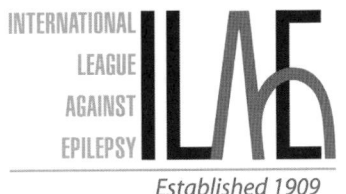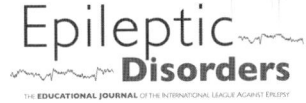

Vol. 21, June 2019 - Supplement 1

Encephalopathy related to Status Epilepticus during slow Sleep: linking epilepsy, sleep disruption and cognitive impairment

Guest Editors:
Guido Rubboli
Carlo Alberto Tassinari

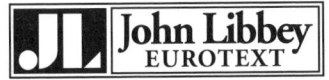

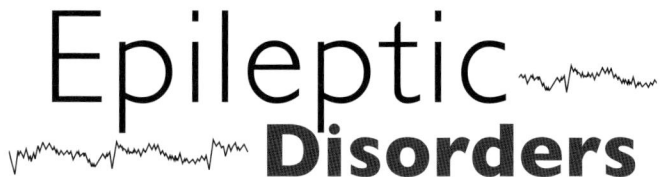

THE EDUCATIONAL JOURNAL OF THE INTERNATIONAL LEAGUE AGAINST EPILEPSY
HTTP://WWW.EPILEPTICDISORDERS.COM

EDITORS-IN-CHIEF

Alexis A. Arzimanoglou
Professor, Epilepsy Research Coordinator,
Hospital Sant Joan de Déu, Universitat de Barcelona, Spain
Head of Department of Paediatric Clinical Epileptology,
Sleep Disorders and Functional Neurology,
University Hospitals of Lyon, France

Sándor Beniczky
Professor, Aarhus University Hospital, Aarhus, Denmark
Head of Clinical Neurophysiology Department, Danish Epilepsy Centre, Dianalund, Denmark

FOUNDING EDITOR

Jean Aicardi
Paris, France

ASSOCIATE EDITORS

Ingmar Blümcke
Erlangen, Germany

Michael Duchowny
Miami, USA

Yushi Inoue
Shizuoka, Japan

Philippe Kahane
Grenoble, France

Rüdiger Köhling
Rostock, Germany

Michalis Koutroumanidis
London, UK

Doug Nordli
Los Angeles, USA

Lieven Lagae
Leuven, Belgium

Guido Rubboli
Dianalund, Denmark

Graeme Sills
Liverpool, UK

Pierre Thomas
Nice, France

Torbjörn Tomson
Stockholm, Sweden

Sarah Wilson
Melbourne, Australia

EDITORIAL BOARD

Nadia Bahi-Buisson
Paris, France

Carmen Barba
Florence, Italy

Fabrice Bartolomei
Marseille, France

Thomas Bast
Kork, Germany

Patricia Braga
Montevideo, Uruguay

Kees Braun
Utrecht, The Netherlands

Roberto Caraballo
Buenos Aires, Argentina

Mar Carreno
Barcelona, Spain

Francine Chassoux
Paris, France

Petia Dimova
Sofia, Bulgaria

David Dunn
Indianapolis, USA

Andras Fogarasi
Budapest, Hungary

Giuseppe Gobbi
Bologna, Italy

Jean Gotman
Montreal, Canada

Gregory Holmes
Vermont, USA

Hans Holthausen
Vogtareuth, Germany

Andres Kanner
Miami, USA

Katsuhiro Kobayashi
Okayama, Japan

Gaetan Lesca
Lyon, France

Shih-Hui Lim
Singapore

Andrew Lux
Bristol, UK

Stefano Meletti
Modena, Italy

Mohamad Mikati
Durham, USA

Fàbio A. Nascimento
Texas, USA

André Palmini
Porto Alegre, Brazil

Georgia Ramantani
Zürich, Switzerland

Aleksandar Ristic
Belgrade, Serbia

Ingrid Scheffer
Melbourne, Australia

Sanjay Sisodiya
London, UK

Mary Lou Smith
Toronto, Canada

Laura Tassi
Milan, Italy

Chong Tin Tan
Kuala Lumpur, Malaysia

Pierangelo Veggiotti
Pavia, Italy

Anna Maria Vezzani
Milan, Italy

Flavio Villani
Milan, Italy

Jo Wilmshurst
Cape Town, South Africa

ILAE EXECUTIVE COMMITTEE

Samuel Wiebe, President
Calgary, Canada

Alla Guekht, Vice President
Moscow, Russian Federation

Edward H. Bertram,
Secretary General
Charlottesville, VA, USA

J. Helen Cross, Treasurer
London, UK

Emilio Perucca, Past President
Pavia, Italy

Angelina Kakooza
Kampala, Uganda

Akio Ikeda
Kyoto, Japan

Eugen Trinka
Salzburg, Austria

Chahnez Triki
Sfax, Tunisia

Roberto Caraballo
Buenos Aires, Argentina

Nathalie Jetté
New York, NY, USA

Astrid Nehlig
Paris, France

Michael Sperling
Philadelphia, PA, USA

Alexis Arzimanoglou
Lyon, France

Aristea Galanopoulou
New York, NY, USA

Shichuo Li
Beijing, China

Nicola Maggio
Tel Aviv, Israel

Xuefeng Wang
Chongqing, China

Jean Gotman
Montreal, Canada

Martin Brodie,
IBE President
Glasgow, Scotland

Mary Secco,
IBE Secretary General
London, Ontario, Canada

Anthony Zimba,
IBE Treasurer
Lusaka, Zambia

EDITORIAL & PRODUCTION STAFF

MANAGING EDITOR
Oliver Gubbay
epileptic.disorders@gmail.com

PUBLICATIONS DIRECTOR
Gilles Cahn
gilles.cahn@jle.com

DESK EDITOR
Marine Rivière
marine.riviere@jle.com

PRODUCT MANAGER
Arnaud Cobo
arnaud.cobo@jle.com

ADVERTISING DIRECTOR
Brigitte Chantrelle
brigitte.chantrelle@jle.com

ISBN: 978-2-7420-1616-7
ISSN: 1294-9361

Published by
Éditions John Libbey Eurotext
127, avenue de la République, 92120 Montrouge, France
Tel.: +33 (0)1 46 73 06 60
www.jle.com

John Libbey Eurotext
42-46 High Street, Esther, Surrey, KT10 9KY
United Kingdom

© 2019, John Libbey Eurotext. All rights reserved.

Unauthorized duplication contravenes applicable laws.
It is prohibited to reproduce this work or any part of it without the authorization of the publisher or of the Centre Français d'Exploitation du Droit de Copie (CFC), 20, rue des Grands-Augustins, 75006 Paris.

Contents

List of authors VII

Preface XI

Linking epilepsy, sleep disruption and cognitive impairment
in Encephalopathy related to Status Epilepticus during slow Sleep (ESES)
    Guido Rubboli, Carlo Alberto Tassinari 1

Encephalopathy related to Status Epilepticus during slow Sleep:
an historical introduction
    Guido Rubboli, Carlo Alberto Tassinari 3

Encephalopathy related to Status Epilepticus during slow Sleep:
from concepts to terminology
    Edouard Hirsch, Roberto Caraballo, Bernardo Dalla Bernardina,
    Tobias Loddenkemper, Sameer M. Zuberi 7

A commentary on Encephalopathy related to Status Epilepticus during slow
Sleep: from concepts to terminology
    Carlo Alberto Tassinari, Guido Rubboli 17

Encephalopathy with continuous spike-waves during slow-wave sleep:
evolution and prognosis
    Roberto Caraballo, Elena Pavlidis, Marina Nikanorova,
    Tobias Loddenkemper 19

EEG features in Encephalopathy related to Status Epilepticus
during slow Sleep
    Elena Gardella, Gaetano Cantalupo, Pål G. Larsson, Elena Fontana,
    Bernardo dalla Bernardina, Guido Rubboli, Francesca Darra 25

Quantitative EEG analysis in Encephalopathy related to Status Epilepticus during slow Sleep
    Gaetano Cantalupo, Elena Pavlidis, Sandor Beniczky, Pietro Avanzini,
    Elena Gardella, Pål G. Larsson 37

Update on the genetics of the epilepsy-aphasia spectrum and role
of GRIN2A mutations
    Gaetan Lesca, Rikke S. Møller, Gabrielle Rudolf, Edouard Hirsch,
    Helle Hjalgrim, Pierre Szepetowski 49

Pathophysiology of encephalopathy related to continuous spike
and waves during sleep: the contribution of neuroimaging
    Michael Siniatchkin, Patrick Van Bogaert 55

Interictal epileptiform discharges in sleep and the role of the thalamus
in Encephalopathy related to Status Epilepticus during slow Sleep
    Steve A. Gibbs, Lino Nobili, Péter Halász 61

Encephalopathy related to Status Epilepticus during slow Sleep:
a link with sleep homeostasis?
    Guido Rubboli, Reto Huber, Giulio Tononi,
    Carlo Alberto Tassinari 69

Cognitive impairment and behavioral disorders in Encephalopathy
related to Status Epilepticus during slow Sleep: diagnostic assessment
and outcome
    Alexis Arzimanoglou, Helen J. Cross 77

Progressive intellectual impairment in children with Encephalopathy
related to Status Epilepticus during slow Sleep
    Liam Dorris, Mary O'Regan, Margaret Wilson,
    Sameer M. Zuberi 83

Current treatment options for Encephalopathy related to Status
Epilepticus during slow Sleep
    Floor E. Jansen, Marina Nikanorova, Maria Peltola 93

Encephalopathy related to Status Epilepticus during slow Sleep:
current concepts and future directions
    Carlo Alberto Tassinari, Guido Rubboli 99

References 105

List of authors

Alexis Arzimanoglou, Department of Paediatric Clinical Epileptology, Sleep Disorders and Functional Neurology, University Hospitals of Lyon (HCL), Member of the European Reference Network EpiCARE, Lyon, France
Epilepsy Unit Hospital San Juan de Dios, Member of the ERN EpiCARE and Universitat de Barcelona, Barcelona, Spain

Pietro Avanzini, Neuroscience Department, University of Parma, Parma, Italy

Sandor Beniczky, Department of Clinical Neurophysiology, Danish Epilepsy Centre, Dianalund University of Aarhus, Aarhus, Denmark

Gaetano Cantalupo, Department of Child Neuropsychiatry, Department of Life and Reproduction Sciences, University of Verona, Italy

Roberto Caraballo, Department of Neurology, Pediatric Hospital Prof. Dr. Juan P Garrahan, Buenos Aires, Argentina

Helen J. Cross, UCL-Great Ormond Street Institute of Child Health, Great Ormond Street Hospital for Children NHS Trust, Member of the European Reference Network EpiCARE, London, UK

Bernardo dalla Bernardina, Department of Child Neuropsychiatry, Department of Life and Reproduction Sciences, University of Verona, Italy

Francesca Darra, Department of Child Neuropsychiatry, Department of Life and Reproduction Sciences, University of Verona, Italy

Liam Dorris, Paediatric Neurosciences Research Group, Royal Hospital for Children
Institute of Health and Wellbeing, University of Glasgow, Member of the European Reference Network EpiCARE, Glasgow, UK

Elena Fontana, Department of Child Neuropsychiatry, Department of Life and Reproduction Sciences, University of Verona, Italy

Elena Gardella, Department of Clinical Neurophysiology, Danish Epilepsy Centre, Dianalund University of Southern Denmark, Odense, Denmark

Steve A. Gibbs, Centre for Epilepsy Surgery "C. Munari", Centre of Sleep Medicine, Department of Neuroscience, Niguarda Hospital, Milan, Italy
Centre for Advanced Studies in Sleep Medicine, Dept. of Neurosciences, Hôpital du Sacré-Coeur de Montreal, Université de Montréal, Montréal, Canada

Peter Halasz, National Institute of Clinical Neuroscience, Budapest, Hungary

Edouard Hirsch, Centre de référence et d'exploration des épilepsies, Pôle Tête Cou / CETD, Neurologie CHU de Strasbourg, Hôpital de Hautepierre, Strasbourg, France
Fédération de Médecine Translationnelle (FMTS), Strasbourg, France
INSERM UMR_SU1119, Strasbourg, France

Helle Hjalgrim, Danish Epilepsy Centre, Dianalund, Denmark
Institute for Regional Health Services, University of Southern Denmark, Odense, Denmark

Reto Huber, Child Development Centre, University Children's Hospital Zurich, Switzerland

Floor E. Jansen, Department of Child Neurology, Brain Center, University medical Center Utrecht, Member of the European Reference Network EpiCARE, The Netherlands
Children's Department, Danish Epilepsy Centre, Dianalund, Denmark

Pal G. Larsson, Department of Neurosurgery, Oslo University Hospital, Oslo, Norway

Gaetan Lesca, Department of Genetics, University Hospitals of Lyon, Member of the European Reference Network EpiCARE Lyon, France
Claude Bernard Lyon I University, Lyon, France
Centre de Recherche en Neurosciences de Lyon, CNRS UMR5292, INSERM U1028, Lyon, France

Tobias Loddenkemper, Division of Epilepsy and Clincial Neurophysiology, Department of Neurology, Boston Children's Hospital, Boston, MA, USA

Rikke S. Møller, Danish Epilepsy Centre, Dianalund, Denmark

Marina Nikanorova, Danish Epilepsy Centre, Dianalund, Denmark

Lino Nobili, Centre for Epilepsy Surgery "C. Munari", Centre of Sleep Medicine, Department of Neuroscience, Niguarda Hospital, Milan, Italy
Child Neuropsychiatry, IRCCS, G. Gaslini Institute, Dept. of Neuroscience (DINOGMI), University of Genoa, Italy

Mary O'Regan, Paediatric Neurosciences Research Group, Royal Hospital for Children, Glasgow, UK

Elena Pavlidis, Child Neuropsychiatry Unit, Neuroscience Department, University of Parma, Italy
Danish Epilepsy Centre, Dianalund, Denmark

Maria Peltola, HUS Medical Imaging Center, Clinical Neurophysiology, University of Helsinki, Helsinki University Hospital and University of Helsinki, Finland

Guido Rubboli, Danish Epilepsy Center, Filadelfia, University of Copenhagen, Dianalund, Denmark

Gabrielle Rudolf, Fédération de Médecine Translationnelle (FMTS), Strasbourg, France
IGBMC, CNRS UMR7104, INSERM U964, Strasbourg University, France
INSERM UMR_SU1119, Strasbourg, France

Michael Siniatchkin, Institute of Medical Psychology and Medical Sociology, Christian-Albrechts-University of Kiel, Germany

Pierre Szepetowski, Aix-Marseille University, INSERM UMR1249, INMED, Marseille, France

Carlo Alberto Tassinari, University of Bologna, Bologna, Italy

Giulio Tononi, Department of Psychiatry, University of Wisconsin, Wisconsin, USA

Patrick Van Bogaert, Department of Pediatric Neurology, CHU d'Angers, and Laboratoire Angevin de Recherche en Ingénierie des Systèmes (LARIS), Université d'Angers, France

Margaret Wilson, Paediatric Neurosciences Research Group, Royal Hospital for Children, Glasgow, UK

Sameer M. Zuberi, Paediatric Neurosciences Research Group, Royal Hospital for Children & University of Glasgow, Member of the European Reference Network EpiCARE, Glasgow, UK

Preface

The interactions between epilepsy, sleep and cognition are complex and reciprocal. Experimental and clinical findings have clearly shown that sleep is beneficial for cognition by actively participating in learning, language acquisition and memory consolidation. These evidences imply that chronic sleep disturbances, particularly in the critical period of brain maturation, may have adverse effects on learning and normal neuropsychological development. In this respect, Encephalopathy related to Status Epilepticus during slow Sleep (ESES), an age-related epileptic syndrome characterized by deterioration of cognitive functions and behavior, epileptic seizures, and extreme activation of EEG epileptiform discharges during non-REM sleep, can represent a privileged model to investigate the deleterious effect of prolonged sleep-related epileptic activity in the developmental age on cognition and behavior. However, in spite of the fact that ESES has been first described almost 50 years ago and that a considerable amount of clinical observations and neurophysiological, neuroimaging, and genetic findings have been accumulated, several issues related to ESES, including the very definition of this condition and its nosology, are still debated and the pathophysiological mechanisms underlying the cognitive and behavioral derangement associated with the appearance of exaggerated sleep-related epileptic activity are poorly understood.

The series of chapters included in this book provides an updated overview on the current knowledge on ESES. Topics such as the clinical and EEG features necessary for the diagnosis, the neurophysiologic and neuropsychological diagnostic assessments, the various therapeutic approaches and the most recent neuroimaging and genetic findings are reviewed with a focus on the most novel aspects. In addition, the fascinating perspectives opened by recent evidences suggesting that the pathophysiological mechanisms underlying the cognitive/behavioral disturbances occurring in ESES might be related to impaired sleep homeostasis caused by prolonged sleep-related epileptic activity are discussed. These latter findings raise the issue that apparently subclinical epileptic activity during sleep might be predicted to have clinical relevance whether appropriately tested (with careful neuropsychological, neuroimaging and neurophysiological testing including also the analysis of EEG parameters assessing sleep homeostasis), not only in ESES but also in larger populations of children with other childhood epilepsies with striking enhancement of epileptic discharges during sleep.

Indeed, we present this book with the intent to identify concepts for which there is a shared view and consolidated knowledge as well as areas where there are still disagreements or controversies and lack of information demanding further studies and research.

This work would have not been possible without the invaluable contribution of the clinicians, neurophysiologists, sleep physiologists and geneticists who have studied ESES and who have taken the burden to contribute their chapters. To them we wish to express our deep appreciation.

Finally, we are very grateful to Prof. Alexis Arzimanoglou at *Epileptic Disorders* for his continuous support and guidance through the manuscript collection and the editing process and to the staff of John Libbey Eurotext for their trademark competence and dedication.

Guido Rubboli, Carlo Alberto Tassinari

Linking epilepsy, sleep disruption and cognitive impairment in Encephalopathy related to Status Epilepticus during slow Sleep (ESES)

Guido Rubboli, Carlo Alberto Tassinari

"Encephalopathy related to Status Epilepticus during slow Sleep (ESES)" was described more than forty-five years ago in a small group of children with learning disabilities who displayed a peculiar EEG pattern consisting of apparently "sub-clinical" spike-and-wave discharges, that occurred almost continuously during sleep for a variable length of time (months to years). Later on, the condition of a protracted "status epilepticus during sleep" (SES) in the developmental age was proposed to be the factor leading to the appearance of severe cognitive and psychic disturbances. Indeed, the extreme activation of epileptic activities during NREM sleep still stands as the electroencephalographic hallmark of a condition that, if prolonged, causes the appearance of a clinical picture that has been acknowledged to be an encephalopathy related to SES. From a broader perspective, SES may be responsible not only for cognitive dysfunctions, such as for instance acquired aphasia, *i.e. Landau-Kleffner syndrome*, but also (and often concomitantly) for other dysfunctions, such as severe behavioral disorders and motor impairment (*i.e.* apraxia and negative myoclonus). Etiology of ESES can be heterogeneous as well, in fact it has been reported in children with organic brain lesions as well as in children with an epilepsy of benign evolution - whether idiopathic or cryptogenic.

After hundreds of observations and comprehensive reviews on the subject (including a monography on the Venice Symposium edited by Beaumanoir *et al.* in 1995), it became clear that SES, cognitive impairment and behavioural disturbances evolve in parallel, and in fact when these latter disorders recover, SES tends to disappear (or it is already over). However, in spite of the wealth of data accumulated over decades, the clinical spectrum of ESES and its boundaries, the diagnostic criteria, the pathophysiology and the therapeutic management are still a matter of debate.

In recent years, clinical observations, neurophysiological and imaging investigations, and genetic studies have renewed interest in ESES. In addition, experimental findings from sleep research have opened fascinating perspectives on some possible pathophysiological mechanisms involved in this condition. These issues have been discussed at the 1st Dianalund International Conference on Epilepsy on *"Encephalopathy related to Status Epilepticus during slow Sleep. Linking epilepsy, sleep disruption and cognitive impairment"* that was organized by Guido Rubboli, Marina Nikanorova, and Carlo Alberto Tassinari on March 14-15, 2014 in Sorø (Denmark). Clinicians, neurophysiologists, sleep physiologists and geneticists (*figure 1*) who have studied ESES gathered with the aim to create a better overall understanding of this special syndrome in the light of recent research. Based on the scientific and educational structure of the meeting, the speakers and session chairs were later invited to contribute with an updated review of their topics. All these contributions are acknowledged in this Supplement with the aim to provide an updated overview of the current knowledge on ESES.

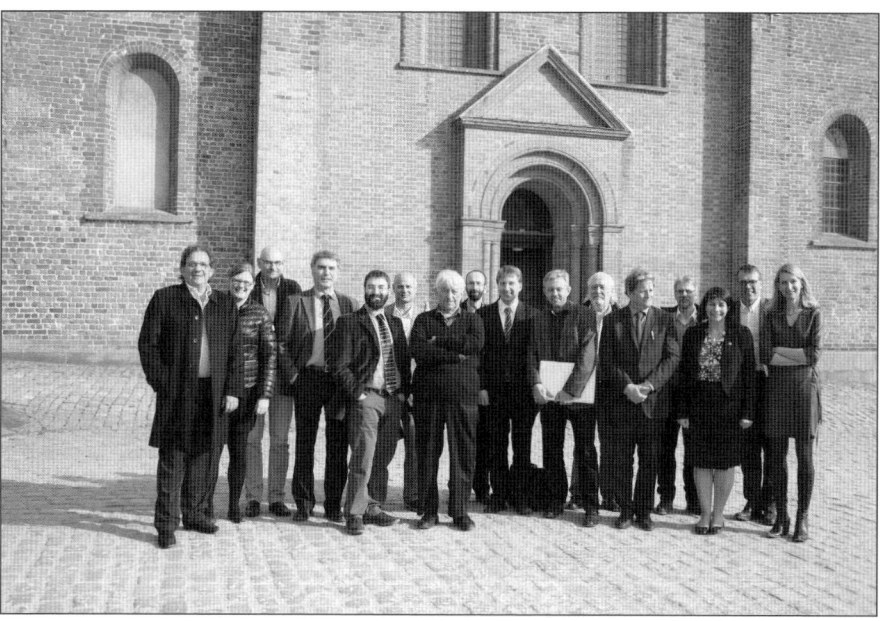

Figure 1/ From left to right: Alexis Arzimanoglou, Rikke S. Møller, José Serratosa, Guido Rubboli, Gaetano Cantalupo, Pierre Szepetowski, Carlo Alberto Tassinari, Sandor Beniczky, Tobias Loddenkemper, Michael Siniatchkin, Philippe Paquier, Edouard Hirsch, Reto Huber, J. Helen Cross, Patrick van Bogaert, Floor E. Jansen.

Encephalopathy related to Status Epilepticus during slow Sleep: an historical introduction

Guido Rubboli, Carlo Alberto Tassinari

In 1971, Patry, Lyagoubi and Tassinari described in six children a distinctive EEG pattern, referred to as "*Subclinical electrical status epilepticus induced by sleep*", characterized by apparently "subclinical" spike-and-wave discharges occurring almost continuously during sleep for a variable length of time (months to years) (figure 1). In 1977, Tassinari et al. reported eleven additional patients. The conclusions of this study (that considered also five of the original patients) stated verbatim: "*the sixteen cases exhibit a peculiar electroclinical syndrome for which the term of Encephalopathy related to Status Epilepticus during slow Sleep, or ESES, is suggested. The EEG shows as soon as the subjects fall asleep, continuous high-voltage diffuse slow spike-and-wave discharges which persist throughout the non-REM sleep. During REM sleep the status epilepticus disappears. Status epilepticus during sleep (SES) can persist for years (up to 8 yrs) and it occurs every time the subjects fall asleep. The waking EEG may or may not show various abnormalities: focal, multifocal, diffuse spikes or spikes and waves. The clinical features can be distinguished into three periods: a) Onset: (4 to 8 yrs) with various types of nocturnal (usually rare) and/or diurnal (atypical absences) seizures present in fifteen cases. One subject never had epileptic seizures. b) Status: characterized by a severe psychic syndrome with psychotic behaviour and mental deterioration. The status period spans from 2 to 8 yrs during which every sleep record*

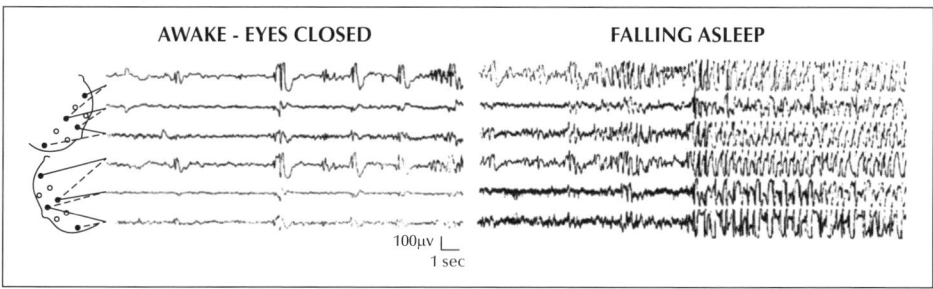

Figure 1/ EEG tracing of an eight-year-old boy showing the transition from wakefulness to sleep and the appearance of continuous spike-and-wave discharge upon falling asleep (modified from the original report by Patry et al., 1971).

shows the status epilepticus. c) Remission: in four cases SES disappeared and the subjects showed progressive improvement in behaviour and mental performances. It is suggested that the condition of a protracted (years) SES can be the factor leading to severe mental deterioration and psychic disturbances in some children. In children with rare seizures and appearance of severe psychic and mental impairment, a sleep record should be considered in search of the ESES ".

As already pointed out (Cantalupo et al., 2013), it is interesting to notice that these conclusions anticipated the concept that was incorporated years later by the International League Against Epilepsy (ILAE) Classification Task Force into the definition of epileptic encephalopathy, including not only the conditions with frequent seizures but also those with a large amount of "interictal" epileptiform activity (Berg et al., 2010).

Kellerman was the first to make the connection between acquired epileptic aphasia, or Landau-Kleffner syndrome (LKS), and extreme activation of spike-and-wave discharges during slow sleep, consistent with SES: *"Landau and Kleffner (1957) suggested that persistence of convulsive discharges in the brain tissue concerned with linguistic communication may result in functional ablation of these areas. This assumption is supported by the report of Patry et al. (1971). Four of their six cases with subclinical sleep-induced bioelectrical status epilepticus have total lack or severe delay of speech. Unfortunately in a supplementary report by one of the authors (Tassinari et al., 1977) no further details are given as to whether the additional patients with subclinical status epilepticus showed evidence of aphasia. However, their children suffered from a severe psychotic syndrome and mental deterioration"* (Kellerman, 1978).

Indeed, in Tassinari's cases (Tassinari et al., 1977), the language impairment was **not** the main clinical feature. Most importantly, in the above citation, Landau and Kleffner referred to epileptic activity during wakefulness and not during sleep. In fact, years later, Landau and Kleffner (2009) commented on sleep-related epileptic activity and LKS: *"Regarding the epilepsy component of LKS, a major constituent of the syndrome of which we had been unaware, is the tremendous exaggeration of paroxysmal brain activity during sleep. We know that such highly abnormal nocturnal EEG are also associated with other clinical syndromes, suggestive of predominant paroxysmal activity in areas other than the auditory territory "*.

In 1989, the International League Against Epilepsy (ILAE) recognized LKS and ESES (otherwise labelled as epilepsy with continuous spike waves during slow-wave sleep - CSWS) as distinct epilepsy syndromes of childhood (whether focal or generalized) (Commission on Classification and Terminology of the International League Against Epilepsy, 1989). However, since the early 2000s, it became accepted that ESES encompassed LKS, this latter representing a clinical variant or subtype of the former (Tassinari et al., 2000). Indeed, the ILAE Task Force in 2006 acknowledged that the current evidence was insufficient to consider LKS and ESES as separate syndromes (Engel, 2006).

One of the most intriguing issues of ESES is the relationship between SES and the pattern of neuropsychological and/or motor impairment. In recent years, numerous experimental data have shown the crucial role of sleep in physiological cognitive and psychomotor development, particularly during the developmental age. Based on these data, it has been hypothesized that prolonged, sleep-related focal epileptic activity interferes with sleep slow wave activity, particularly at the site of the epileptic focus, hence disrupting the cortical plasticity processes occurring during sleep that are necessary for learning and memory consolidation of what has been acquired in wakefulness, ultimately resulting in neuropsychological and behavioural disorders (Tassinari and Rubboli, 2006). In fact, some recent reports support this hypothesis, by providing electrophysiological evidence that physiological parameters related to NREM slow-wave activity are impaired in children with ESES and recover after ESES resolution (Bölsterli *et al.*, 2011, 2017). These concepts, that provide a fascinating pathophysiological explanation linking the cognitive impairment to the sleep-related exaggerated epileptic activity that characterize ESES, are efficaciously conveyed by the eponym "Penelope syndrome" in which the 'cognitive threads' (neuronal networks) that are weaved during the day are unravelled (by continuous "spiking") during the night (Tassinari *et al.*, 2009).

Encephalopathy related to Status Epilepticus during slow Sleep: from concepts to terminology

Edouard Hirsch, Roberto Caraballo, Bernardo Dalla Bernardina, Tobias Loddenkemper, Sameer M. Zuberi

Despite Encephalopathy related to Status Epilepticus during slow Sleep (ESES) being first reported more than 45 years ago, its defining features and diagnostic criteria are still a matter of debate. In addition, inconsistent terminology and concepts are used when referring to ESES, possibly causing unnecessary difficulties in the delineation of the syndrome and in the interpretation of the results provided by different studies. Edouard Hirsch, Roberto Caraballo, Bernardo Dalla Bernardina, Tobias Loddenkemper and Sameer M. Zuberi, five "epileptologists" with interest and experience in the diagnosis and management of ESES, express their opinions on the definition, the diagnostic assessment and the terminology that may be considered for this condition by answering selected predefined questions. The aim is to identify concepts for which there is a shared view (such as, for instance, ESES as a childhood epileptic encephalopathy encompassing Landau-Kleffner syndrome; the need to demonstrate, for the diagnosis of ESES, that the sleep EEG pattern has a clinical correlate, that is the appearance of cognitive/behavioral disorders; the possible role of disruption of sleep homeostasis), and areas where there are still disagreements on classification or controversies (such as, for instance, EEG evaluation and biomarkers, neuropsychological assessment, and terminology) which demand further studies and research (see also Tassinari and Rubboli, p. 99-103).

1) Is ESES a syndrome or a "self-limited" EEG pattern like hypsarrhythmia?

Roberto Caraballo (RC). It is an epileptic syndrome within the group of epileptic encephalopathies. According to age at onset, clinical manifestations, EEG pattern, evolution and prognosis, independent of etiology, it meets the criteria of the well-defined epileptic syndrome (Commission ILAE, 1989).

Bernardo Dalla Bernardina (BDB). ESES and Landau Kleffner syndrome (LKS) are one syndrome with variable clinical features; it is a childhood-onset encephalopathy characterized by the appearance of neuropsychological and behavioral disorders related to a significant and sustained activation of EEG paroxysms from drowsiness throughout all NREM sleep.

The clinical impairment can appear abruptly or progressively:
- it can appear in a previously normal child or it can be a worsening of a pre-existing neuropsychological impairment;
- it can be a global cognitive impairment or it can concern a specific domain only (Kuki et al., 2014);
- the behavioral and psychiatric disorders can be of variable type and degree, leading to an autistic-like condition in some cases.

This peculiar electroclinical condition can appear, for unknown reasons (genetic predisposition, immunological mechanism, etc.), in any type of focal epilepsy of infancy or childhood of genetic (idiopathic), structural (both genetic or acquired), or unknown origin (Dalla Bernardina et al., 1978, 1989). In some cases, it can be induced by some AEDs.

Even if the mechanisms inducing the impairment are probably multiple and complex, one important factor can be a focal (Huber et al., 2004) or diffuse (Tononi and Cirelli 2014) disruption of sleep homeostasis induced by the recurrence of paroxysms (Tassinari and Rubboli, 2006; Cantalupo et al., 2011).

Edouard Hirsch (EH). Syndromes are defined according to non-fortuitous associations with signs and symptoms. To date, syndrome definitions have been based on expert opinions. In 2014, an ILAE position paper (Fisher et al., 2014) recognized epilepsies and syndromes as a group of diseases. The 1989 classification of epilepsies was revised in 2017 (Scheffer et al., 2017) (figure 1).

The Nosology and Definition Task force of the ILAE in 2018 are still discussing the definition of a syndrome. It is proposed that a syndrome is a characteristic cluster of clinical, EEG and laboratory (imaging, neuropsychology, etc.) features in an individual with epilepsy, often with etiologic, prognostic and therapeutic implications. Syndromes may have age-dependent presentations and specific co-morbidities.

The main changes in classification for "LKS"- "ESES" are presented in (figure 2):
- Epilepsy Type: Generalized and Focal seizures may co-exist;
- "LKS"-"ESES", may have multiple etiologies even in an individual patient eg. genetic, structural, immune, inflammatory, metabolic.

The new ILAE commission on classification and terminology "2017-2021" is going to work on "syndrome" definitions and limits. One of the difficulties for this new commission is to try to have a scientific-based definition of syndromes.

Until now, I personally think that:

LKS and ESES are one syndrome: *Childhood-onset Epileptic Encephalopathy with usually Generalized and/or Focal seizures and always Cognitive and Behavioral Acquired Co-morbidities and a Self-limited EEG pattern characterized by activation of Focal and Generalized EEG pathological "epileptiform transients" during sleep responsible for disruption of Sleep Homeostasis**.

* Disruption of sleep homeostasis: location and density of spike waves and slow waves are related to an alteration of the physiologic overnight decrease of the focal slow wave slope (Hirsch et al 2006; Bölsterli Heinzle et al 2014; see also Rubboli et al., p. 69-76).

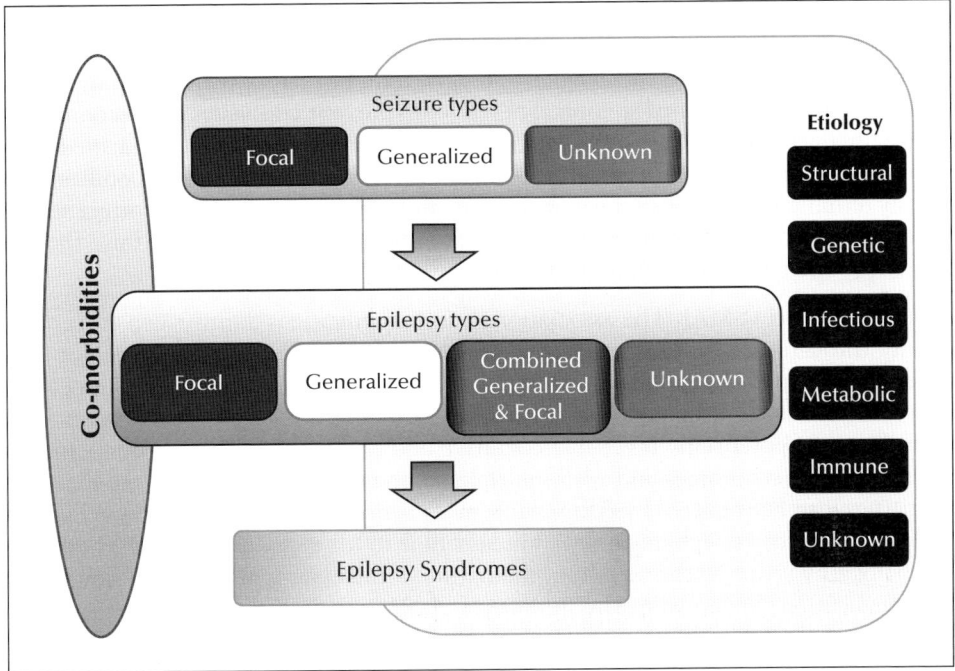

Figure 1/ 2017 classification of epilepsies.

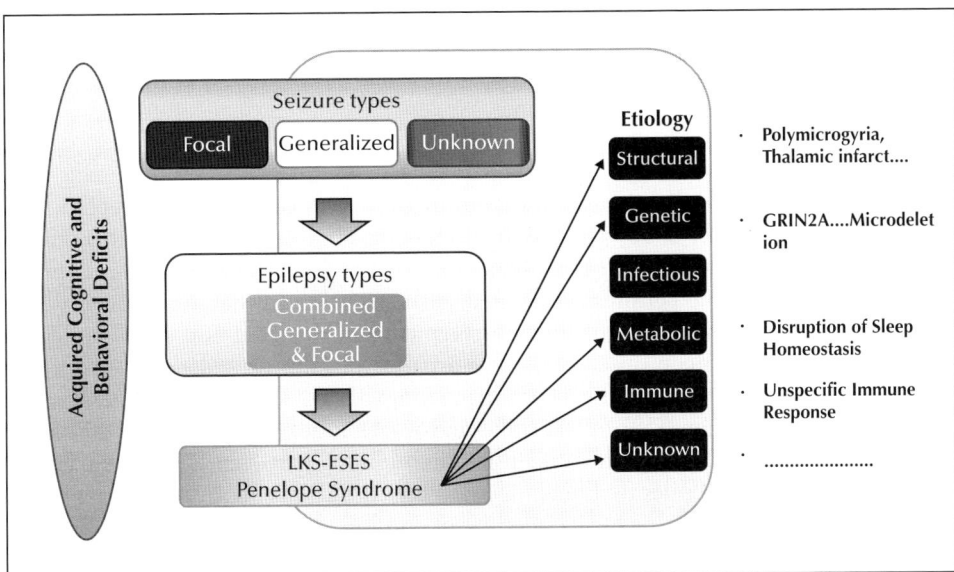

Figure 2/ LKS-ESES etiologies.

Tobias Loddenkemper (TL). Physicians utilize ESES terminology differently, and this may lead to miscommunication (Fernandez et al., 2013). Due to lack of consistent use, several colleagues conferred, and decided to use the term ESES for the EEG finding of sleep-potentiated or sleep-activated spiking. Therefore, to prevent confusion or miscommunication, we usually use ESES to describe the EEG feature that is one of the diagnostic features for epileptic encephalopathies within this seizure susceptibility complex of conditions. As with any terminology, this is simply convention, and there is ultimately no correct solution one way or another, as this is simply a term. However, it is crucial that all use the same terminology and assessment approach (Fernandez et al., 2013).

Sameer M. Zuberi (SMZ). The association of status epilepticus during sleep and encephalopathy through childhood is associated with too many different aetiologies, too many different treatments and too many different outcomes for it to be classified as an epilepsy syndrome. ESES should be regarded as an important self-limited EEG pattern associated with a degree of potentially reversible cognitive and physical impairment that can occur in many epilepsy syndromes and with multiple different aetiologies. As noted above, this EEG pattern can be triggered by AEDs. How many syndromes are produced by AEDs? The broader concept of encephalopathy is fundamental to all types of epilepsy, whether the encephalopathy is due to the aetiology, the nature of the epilepsy type or syndrome or the use of medication. Encephalopathy in epilepsy should not be separated into a syndrome. The potential for different degrees of encephalopathy must be acknowledged in everyone with the brain disease epilepsy and having a separate group "the epileptic encephalopathies" averts the gaze of the clinician to this important issue.

Epilepsy classification should serve better treatments and encourage research in the epilepsies. Clinical groupings comprising many conditions with shared EEG features but markedly disparate aetiologies, outcomes and treatments such as Ohtahara syndrome, Lennox-Gastaut syndrome and ESES have had an important role in the history of epilepsy classification but have reduced clinical relevance as science reveals underlying aetiologies and mechanisms with the goal of more precise therapies (Scheffer, 2017).

Landau-Kleffner syndrome (LKS) is an epilepsy in which ESES is a key clinical feature and I would regard LKS as an epilepsy syndrome.

2) If it is a syndrome, what are the minimum criteria for definition?

RC. This is a well-defined epileptic syndrome in the group of epileptic encephalopathy (Engel, 2001: Berg et al., 2010) starting in childhood characterized by focal motor seizures, complex focal seizures, apparently generalized seizures (clonic, tonic-clonic seizures, absences), and myoclonic seizures, associated with neurological deterioration involving cognitive, behavioral and/or motor domains. Typical EEG pattern is a status epilepticus during sleep (ESES) at sleep onset defined as a pattern of diffuse spike-and-waves (symmetric, asymmetric, unilateral or focal) occurring in up 85% of slow sleep and persisting for months or years. Less than 85% of the spike-and-waves index should also be considered. Its relationship with focal idiopathic epilepsies of childhood particularly Rolandic epilepsy is very well known, and Epileptic Encephalopathy with SES may correspond to a broader clinical phenotype of idiopathic focal epilepsies of childhood. The genetic findings in these groups of patients could be explained by their close genetic link. Landau-Kleffner syndrome could be considered a variant of Epileptic Encephalopathy with SES considering that most of the patients with auditory verbal agnosia present ESES.

BDB. (A) Childhood onset; (B) appearance or worsening of Neuropsychological and/or Cognitive and/or Behavioral impairment; (C) Self-limited EEG pattern characterized by sustained focal and/or diffuse EEG paroxysms activated by drowsiness throughout all NREM sleep; (D) Focal/multifocal/generalized seizures mainly nocturnal, and rare in most cases. In some cases overt clinical seizures may be lacking; (E) Atypical absences with or without associated motor phenomena, mainly inhibitory, in some cases.

Only A,B,C are consequently mandatory criteria.

EH. (A) Childhood onset; (B) Cognitive and Behavioral Acquired impairment; (C) Self-limited EEG pattern characterized by activation of Focal and Generalized EEG pathological "epileptiform transients" during Sleep responsible of Sleep Homeostasis Disruption; (D) Generalized and/or Focal seizures

Mandatory: A+B+C

TL. ESES may refer to the EEG pattern associated with childhood seizure susceptibility syndromes, including Landau Kleffner syndrome, and Continuous Spike and Wave during Slow wave sleep (CSWS). For a suspected diagnosis of CSWS, consideration of the following parameters may be helpful: A) childhood onset, B) sleep-potentiated/-activated generalized or focal spiking or sharp waves, C) comorbidities in two cognitive/developmental domains (including fine and gross motor, language and social/behavioral, among others), and - not mandatorily - generalized and/or focal epileptic seizures. For a suspected diagnosis of LKS, consideration of the following parameters may be helpful: A) childhood onset, B) sleep-potentiated/-activated generalized/focal spiking or sharp waves on EEG and C) impairment in language development, and - not mandatorily - generalized and/or focal epileptic seizures.

Ultimately, a longitudinal course, recognition of evolution through different disease stages (Fernández et al., 2012), and application of treatment and response to treatment (specifically in EEG and cognitive features) may also serve as confirmation of a diagnosis. Response to treatment may be more evident in children presenting with more frequent spiking and more acute or more severe onset of development and cognitive features, or lesser cognitive reserve, including regression. Therefore, response to treatment and resolution over time may be an additional diagnostic criterion, and while confirmatory, this approach may at times not be practical when encountering a patient during the acute phase of the condition. However, a similar approach including the response to intervention has been successfully adopted for non-convulsive status epilepticus (Beniczky et al., 2013).

SMZ. As described above, I do not regard ESES as a separate syndrome. I would agree that the features of ESES include: A. Childhood onset; B. Encephalopathy with acquired impairment of cognitive, behavioral and sometimes motor function; C. Self-limited focal and generalized spike-wave EEG abnormalities during sleep sufficient to disrupt sleep homeostasis.

These criteria are insufficient in themselves to comprise a syndrome. The disruption to sleep homeostasis and the functions of sleep is critical to understanding the impact of status epilepticus during sleep. Sleep is for the brain and generated by the brain. Understanding how sleep disruption in general impacts on health and well-being in epilepsy is an important focus of research. Normal sleep is required for memory and learning with increasing evidence that consciousness and the organization and encoding of long-term memories are mutually exclusive. We need to undertake these processes in sleep in order to allow us to have reference points for consciousness in wakefulness.

3) Which EEG diagnostic criteria would you endorse for the diagnosis of ESES?

RC. We believe that the definition of the electro-clinical inclusion criteria of the epileptic syndrome or epilepsy type is fundamental, however accepting very strict inclusion criteria may sometimes hinder the inclusion of patients with typical or classical EEG patterns. Thus, we think that a group of patients with the characteristic clinical manifestation of epileptic encephalopathy but less than 85% of the ESES (between 50 to 85%) should be included. Other types of EEG abnormalities during slow sleep, such as multifocal spikes, frequent asynchronous bilateral spikes, diffuse slow-wave activity and different morphology of EEG abnormalities in both cerebral hemispheres should also be considered and discussed in the EEG inclusion criteria (Caraballo et al., 2015).

One point is to define the quantitative and qualitative EEG parameters in our daily practice and which are the EEG parameters that we should consider methodologically to develop a scientific study. A sleep EEG recording lasting 30-60 minutes could be enough in the first situation, whereas a whole-night NREM sleep should be considered in the second. There are different proposals to define the qualitative and quantitative aspect of ESES (see also Gardella et al., p. 25-36), thus a consensus should be crucial to delineate the EEG inclusion criteria for this syndrome considering also the facilities commonly available in neurological departments.

BDB. The only EEG criterion is constituted by a sustained activation of focal and/or diffuse EEG paroxysms from drowsiness throughout all NREM sleep, provided that it is related to a documented clinical impairment.

The paroxysms can remain focal (unilateral or bilateral) (see *figure 3* in Gardella et al., p. 22-30 hemispheric (see *figure 4* in Gardella et al., p. 25-36) or they can become bilaterally diffuse (see *figures 1, 2* in Gardella et al., p. 25-36).

The frequency of the paroxysms is not part of the definition but they must be clearly and continuously more frequent than during wakefulness.

Even if frequency, topography, and morphology of the EEG paroxysms do not constitute diagnostic criteria, they must nevertheless be analyzed and reported because the clinical features can vary according to different EEG patterns.

On awakening, the paroxysms can be focal/multifocal/diffuse or, although rarely, even absent. Consequently, EEG paroxysms on awakening do not constitute a mandatory criterion.

EH. Self-limited EEG pattern characterized by the following:

1 During wakefulness: focal and/or generalized focal or multifocal spikes and/or spike-waves; "epileptiform transient"

2 Tangential dipole for "epileptiform transient"

3 Sleep activation of focal and/or generalized EEG transients

Mandatory: 1+2+3

TL. A) Sleep-activated/-potentiated focal or generalized spikes and sharp waves are supportive of a diagnosis, specifically during sleep stages I, II, and III. Spikes and sharp waves may be generalized or focal (Fernández et al., 2013; see also Gardella et al., p. 25-36). These spikes and sharp waves are usually not seen at the same frequency during wakefulness or REM sleep. While the spike-wave index and spike frequencies during slow-wave sleep are most frequently used, ranging from 25% to 100% (or with even greater range), and while a spike wave index of at least 50% may be overall helpful, a specific cut off may not be the optimal EEG parameter, depending on the stage of the condition, as EEGs are at this point merely reflective of a short period of time, and based on assessment method. Of note, the spike wave index may temporarily drop below any certain percentage during treatment, and recur, but this drop does not imply that the condition has entirely resolved, and may likely imply sampling and information bias. Equally important for diagnosis rather than the actual frequency of spiking during sleep may also be the sleep (including stages I, II, and III) to wakefulness (or REM) ratio of spikes, meaning that spikes usually are more frequent during sleep than during wakefulness, and a ratio greater than 3:1 may frequently suggest a diagnosis. Again, this marker also suffers from sampling and information bias. Please note that any of these cut-off ratios have limitations, and that a combination of overall sleep frequency and a ratio between sleep and wakefulness over time may be most helpful. Ultimately, any specific figures for spike frequency/spike wave index, or a spike ratio may be based on expert opinion, and while currently most practical, both may only be a placeholder for more improved detailed longitudinal EEG assessments in the future.

B) Disruption or lack of normal sleep features and patterns may also help with the diagnosis. As outlined, spike frequency or spike wave index can be relatively conveniently assessed. Other EEG biomarkers, such as a lack of or decrease in normal sleep features, such as spindles, Vertex waves, and K-complexes, as well as disruption of sleep cycling, high-frequency in relation to slowing, and a related lack of changes in the slope of the slow wave sleep throughout the night, among others, may ultimately prove to be better EEG biomarkers (see also Rubboli et al., p. 69-76, and Tassinari and Rubboli, p. 99-103). A simple biomarker, until better tools are available for assessment, without calculation of the slow-wave sleep slope over time, may be lack of (or reduction of) normal sleep features, implying also disruption of sleep homeostasis and nighttime memory formation and learning.

SMZ. Duration of the status epilepticus in sleep will impact on the degree of sleep homeostasis disruption however the duration required to produce an acquired encephalopathy will vary from individual to individual. Setting this percentage at 85%, 50% or 30% is to a degree arbitrary. The term *status* in epilepsy implies a particular continuous duration of focal or generalized EEG discharges or clinical abnormalities. The abnormalities in ESES may not be continuous throughout slow wave sleep.

Whether a particular percentage of sleep disruption results in an acquired cognitive, behavioral or motor impairment will depend on the resilience of the individual brain influenced by many factors (genetic and environmental) and also on the sensitivity of measures assessing impairment. The presence of spike-wave abnormalities in the awake EEG is not required.

ESES is present when there is a measurable acquired encephalopathy (cognitive, behavioral, +/- motor impairment) associated with sleep activation of focal and generalized spike-wave abnormalities.

4) How do you assess the occurrence of Encephalopathy in SES?

RC. By definition, neurological deterioration occurs in all cases of this syndrome. It usually is coincidental with the detection of ESES representing one of the crucial signs of the syndrome. The encephalopathy is represented most frequently by a combination of disturbances in one or more domains, including language, cognition, behavior, and motor abilities. A neuropsychological and motor assessment follow-up in all patients is fundamental to define neurological deterioration, their relationship with ESES, response to the treatment, evolution and prognosis. According to the cognitive profile of the patients we should choose the neuropsychological test to perform (see also Arzimanoglou and Cross, p. 77-81).

BDB. Considering that the diagnosis of ESES requires that the abnormal increase of the EEG paroxysms during sleep is associated with a documented appearance or worsening of a clinical impairment, the diagnosis and the management of ESES needs both repeated sleep EEG and neuropsychological assessments.

In the case in which the abnormal increase of the EEG paroxysms during sleep appears or is recognized in a child for whom a previous adequate neuropsychological assessment is available, the diagnosis of ESES can be done if a new assessment documents a neuropsychological impairment.

If a previous neuropsychological assessment is lacking, the diagnosis of ESES can be done if two sleep EEG-neuropsychological assessments (separated by 1-3 months) document a progressive impairment. The interval must be chosen according to the clinical picture.

The diagnosis of ESES can be ascertained upon recognition of the EEG picture during sleep in cases in which the sleep EEG has been performed due to the appearance of an unexplained clinical impairment.

EH. Onset of cognitive and/or behavioral acquired impairment not related to AEDs.

TL. Cognitive and behavioral co-morbidities in language, fine and gross motor, or social/behavioral domains, among others, play a role. Presence of regression (loss of function in different domains) is most significant, but may not always be present, depending on the stage of the condition and depending on prior treatment. Cognitive findings should ideally not be easily explained by other etiologies.

SMZ. The encephalopathy is the clinical impairment and as such ESES cannot be defined on EEG criteria alone. It is important that children with ESES have early and continuing neuropsychological assessment and that developmental monitoring is linked with appropriate psychological, social and psychiatric support to improve mental wellbeing and social participation. Evaluations need to be consistent in any individual and separated by a reasonable time. Re-testing using the same neuropsychological instrument may require a gap of 6 months. General observation and description of behaviour does have clinical value and should not be neglected. Full scale IQ and performance IQ should be evaluated with awareness that more specific impairments in subsets including verbal IQ may be present (Dorris et al., p. 83-92). Instruments for behavioral assessment such as the Child Behavior Checklist (CBCL) should be considered. If motor impairments develop alongside cognitive and behavioral problems, these should also be assessed including the use of serial videotape recordings.

5) How would you define the resolution of ESES?

BDB. A recovery or a documented improvement of the neuropsychological picture related to the disappearance of the abnormal activation of EEG paroxysms during sleep.

The improvement can be transient or permanent. Only with an adequate follow-up according to the age of the child can resolution be considered as permanent.

In several cases, the clinical improvement following the EEG improvement can be very slow and in many cases, it is not a complete recovery. Consequently, the resolution of ESES must be considered as the resolution of the EEG picture associated with a clinical improvement and not necessarily the recovery of the pre-ESES clinical status.

EH. Recovery of pre-morbid cognitive and/or behavioral status.

TL. With regards to resolution of the condition, recovery of EEG biomarkers and neurodevelopmental features to baseline levels (or ideally levels relative to normal peers at the same age) for extended periods of time (ideally into adulthood) may be optimal, and resolution of seizures may be supportive. However, depending on etiology, some patients may have life-long cognitive deficits and continue to present with EEG features later in life, and with current monitoring and interventions may not return to premorbid or peer-related baseline. Remission of EEG features may be defined by reduction of EEG features below diagnostic criteria, but similar to other conditions, frequent monitoring may be required into adulthood to evaluate for recurrence.

SMZ. The disappearance or significant improvement in the EEG abnormalities with no further evidence of a progressive encephalopathy as demonstrated by neuropsychological assessment. Many of the children after resolution of the ESES do not return to their premorbid state (Dorris et al., p. 83-92).

6) Several eponyms have been proposed, *i.e.* ESES (encephalopathy related to status epilepticus during slow sleep), CSWS (continuous spike and waves during sleep), ECSWS (encephalopathy with continuous spike and waves during sleep), Tassinari's syndrome. Is there one that you would suggest, or would you propose an alternative one?

BDB. In my opinion the best choice would be *"Tassinari's syndrome"*. If the introduction of new eponyms is no longer accepted by the ILAE Classification Task Force, the only choice justified is "ESES", *i.e.* "Encephalopathy related to Status Epilepticus during slow Sleep".

For the syndrome definition, the term CSWS is unacceptable because it is an EEG descriptor and it is impossible to define a syndrome on the basis of the EEG pattern only. However, the EEG pattern cannot be described using the term of the syndrome. Hypsarrhythmia is not a syndrome and West syndrome is not a descriptor of the hypsarrhythmic pattern.

The term CSWS may be used to describe the EEG pattern. The criticism of this choice would be the fact that the component "continuous" is not mandatory in the definition of the syndrome. One possibility would be to describe the condition as "Spike Wave Status during Sleep" (SWSS).

In other words, ESES (Encephalopathy related to Status Epilepticus during Sleep) is in fact an epileptic "Encephalopathy with SW Status during Sleep, *i.e.* ESWSS".

LKS is one of the clinical types of ESES with predominant language impairment as well as cases with "autistic regression", cases with "absences and inhibitory phenomena", "atypical benign partial epilepsies (ABPE)", and cases with "specific neuropsychological impairment". These latter conditions are other clinical types of ESES needing in some way different treatments and especially different rehabilitative strategies.

EH. Current 1989 definitions for LKS as well as for ESES are too narrow. Former ILAE Classification Commissions & Task Forces do not seem to support new eponyms for syndromes. One alternative is Penelope Syndrome of Childhood (PSC) to name a Self-Limited Childhood Epileptic Encephalopathy with Spike Wave Status during Sleep and disruption of sleep homeostasis (Cantalupo et al., p. 37-48).

TL. It is crucial recognize the ground-breaking contributions of Drs. Tassinari, Landau, and Kleffner, and many others, also including the prestigious coauthors of this article and in this special issue, to the spectrum of these conditions, and I would like to honor the contributions of these pioneers in the field. However, allow me to also recognize that any specific terminology may not be sufficiently broad to capture the longitudinal presentation and evolution as well as implications of this spectrum of conditions for learning, memory and development during sleep. An overarching terminology for the spectrum of these conditions would be very helpful, and some colleagues currently try to broadly refer to this larger category as childhood seizure susceptibility syndrome(s), in an attempt to characterize the longitudinal course as well as temporary susceptibility to increased epileptogenicity and often temporary sleep features and pattern disruption. While there is need for a common broader term, there are no scientific arguments for or against certain terminology, only expert opinion. A common terminology would, however, greatly benefit all, most importantly including our patients, and facilitate recognition, care, treatment, and future research.

SMZ. Encephalopathy related to Status Epilepticus during slow Sleep (ESES) includes the key clinical features and is sufficient. As I don't regard the clinical entity as consistent enough to be a syndrome, I don't think it should be given an eponymous name.

Landau-Kleffner syndrome is appropriate for this condition.

A commentary on Encephalopathy related to Status Epilepticus during slow Sleep: from concepts to terminology

Carlo Alberto Tassinari, Guido Rubboli

The "debate" among Edouard Hirsch, Roberto Caraballo, Bernardo Dalla Bernardina, Tobias Loddenkemper and Sameer Zuberi (Hirsch et al., p. 7-16) highlights effectively some shared concepts that define Encephalopathy related to Status Epilepticus during slow Sleep (ESES). There is a large consensus among the five experts that the cardinal features that characterize ESES are: a) childhood onset; b) self-limited focal or generalized enhancement of EEG abnormalities during NREM sleep; c) acquired impairment of cognitive, behavioral and sometimes motor functions related to the appearance of the peculiar sleep EEG pattern; epileptic seizures are almost always present but their occurrence is not mandatory for the diagnosis of ESES.

We and most of the experts that participated in the debate believe that the three main features listed above can indeed define ESES as a separate syndrome with its nosographic place within the group of epileptic encephalopathies (see also Tassinari and Rubboli, p. 99-103).

This opinion is supported by the evidence of children, neurologically and cognitively normal before ESES onset (*i.e.*, with idiopathic etiology), who start to present with cognitive and behavioral deterioration in concomitance with a striking exaggeration of EEG epileptic activity during NREM sleep (*i.e.* "status epilepticus during sleep (SES)"), without evidence of other factors that can derange neuropsychological development and regardless of the presence of diurnal or nocturnal epileptic seizures.

We believe that **idiopathic ESES** is a specific condition, which in some cases represents the evolution of an idiopathic rolandic epilepsy, but in other cases represents a condition in its own right from onset (patients presenting with seizures other than rolandic seizures, or even no seizures at all), and it illustrates the "core" concept of ESES itself, that is the deleterious, sometimes permanent, effects on cognitive/behavioral functions associated with exaggerated epileptic activity during NREM sleep in the developmental age.

From this perspective, LKS (which by definition does not have a symptomatic etiology) indeed appears to be a variant of idiopathic ESES, with a well defined neuropsychological deficit (auditory agnosia and language impairment). Once more, we wish to point out that the concept of the harmful effect of epileptic activity "*per se*" is incorporated into the definition of epileptic encephalopathy by the International League Against Epilepsy (ILAE) Classification Task Force (Berg *et al.*, 2010), which includes not only conditions with frequent seizures but also those with a large amount of "interictal" epileptiform activity. In addition, in agreement with the recent ILAE proposals on the definition of "syndrome" (Berg et al., 2010; Scheffer et al., 2017), we believe that ESES is a syndrome defined by specific electro-clinical features, independent of etiology and indeed, can be associated with different etiologies.

It can be hypothesized that the striking enhancement of epileptic activity during NREM sleep (due to a structural etiology, antiepileptic drugs, or other factors?), that can occur in etiologically heterogeneous conditions, may disrupt sleep-related consolidation and maturation of cognitive processes, resulting in or aggravating an encephalopathy, involving pathogenetic mechanisms similar to those underlying "idiopathic" ESES.

We consider "status epilepticus during sleep" in ESES as a clinical condition characterized by sustained and protracted epileptic activity. As in other types of status epilepticus in which it is not necessary to quantify the amount of epileptic spikes to diagnose the status itself, but it is the electro-clinical picture that orients the diagnosis, we wish to tone down the relevance that has been given to the spike-wave index (SWI) in the diagnosis of ESES since its first description (Patry et al., 1971). The SWI threshold to diagnose ESES can be flexible, and can be <85%, provided that the main feature of ESES, *i.e.* occurrence of cognitive and behavioral deterioration associated with a striking enhancement of epileptic activity during NREM sleep, is demonstrated.

These latter considerations raise the issue of other sleep-related parameters, besides SWI, that can play a pathogenetic role in ESES. We and all the experts agree that a derangement of sleep homeostasis caused by the exaggerated epileptic discharges during NREM sleep might play a crucial role in ESES. In recent years, a wealth of experimental and clinical research on sleep physiology has shown the important role of sleep homeostasis in memory consolidation and in learning processes (Tononi and Cirelli, 2014). Recently, some studies have shown that an impairment of sleep homeostasis caused by sleep-related epileptic activity could play a role in the cognitive derangement of ESES (Bolsterli et al., 2011, 2014, 2017; Rubboli et al., p. 69-76; Tassinari and Rubboli, p. 99-103). We wish to emphasize the relevance of these findings to better understand ESES pathophysiology, but also because of the possible implications in the management of other epileptic conditions with a striking increment of epileptic activity during sleep in the developmental age.

In conclusion, in our opinion, what qualifies ESES as a unique and identifiable condition, *i.e.* a syndrome, is not just the peculiar EEG picture of the striking exaggeration of epileptic discharges during sleep, which can be subtended by different etiologies, but the dramatic, and often irreversible effects that this sleep-related epileptic activity can produce in developmental age on cognition and behavior. Several recent data suggest that sleep-related derangement of sleep homeostasis caused by protracted epileptic activity during sleep might be responsible for the encephalopathic picture. In this respect, ESES is a privileged model for the investigation of the reciprocal interactions between epilepsy, sleep and cognition.

Encephalopathy with continuous spike-waves during slow-wave sleep: evolution and prognosis

Roberto Caraballo, Elena Pavlidis, Marina Nikanorova, Tobias Loddenkemper

■ Definition and nosological aspects

Encephalopathy with continuous spike-waves during slow-wave sleep (CSWS) is an age-related syndrome characterized by neurocognitive regression, seizures, and an EEG pattern of electrical status epilepticus during sleep. Onset of the CSWS syndrome is typically between the ages of 4 and 7 years with seizures accompanied by developmental regression. The syndrome sometimes presents in children beyond the age of 10-12 years and cases as young as two years of age have been reported (Bureau, 1995; Loddenkemper et al., 2011). CSWS presents in children with structural or metabolic epilepsy associated with different types of brain lesions, it may be related to genetic or probably genetic causes, or the etiology may be unknown. The syndrome may be diagnosed when CSWS occurs in more than 85% of non-REM sleep; however, the classification of the ILAE does not specify a cut-off value (Commission on Classification and Terminology of the International League Against Epilepsy, 1989).

Although the pattern of CSWS is the main diagnostic criterion of the CSWS syndrome, it is also observed in other syndromes that are now considered to be part of the same clinical spectrum, including atypical benign partial epilepsy of childhood (ABPEC), status of benign childhood epilepsy with centrotemporal spikes (SEBCECTS), and Landau-Kleffner syndrome (LKS) (Fejerman et al., 2000; Loddenkemper et al., 2011). All four conditions have been reported as atypical evolutions in children with a previous diagnosis of benign childhood epilepsy with centrotemporal spikes (BCECTS) (Fejerman et al., 2000). Patients with BCECTS may also evolve to a so-called "mixed form of atypical evolutions" showing the CSWS pattern associated with clinical features of ABPEC, SEBCECTS, LKS, and typical CSWS (Fejerman et al., 2000). Additionally, an atypical evolution associated with CSWS has been reported in children with Panayiotopoulos syndrome and in those with childhood epilepsy with occipital paroxysms of Gastaut (Caraballo et al., 2001, 2011).

Landau-Kleffner syndrome shares many clinical and EEG features with the CSWS syndrome; however, in the former it is more often associated with acquired aphasia while in the latter psychiatric disturbances are more commonly found (Tassinari *et al.*, 2000).

CSWS may occur in children with organic brain lesions, of which unilateral polymicrogyria (PMG) is the most common (Caraballo *et al.*, 2013a, 2013b), and shunted hydrocephalus, indicative of thalamo-cortical circuitries (Veggiotti *et al.*, 1998; Caraballo *et al.*, 1999, 2008; Ben-Zeev *et al.*, 2004).

■ Evolution

CSWS evolves over time, and modifications of clinical seizures, EEG abnormalities, and neurocognition occur. Three stages have been reported (Sánchez Fernández *et al.*, 2012).

In the first stage, before the onset of CSWS, patients often show infrequent nocturnal motor focal seizures: in addition, hemiclonic status epilepticus, absences, atonic, complex focal seizures, and generalized tonic-clonic seizures can often occur. Age at epilepsy onset in the pre-CSWS period peaks between four and five years (range: 2-12 years). In this stage, abnormal EEG findings are observed that always include potentiation of spiking during non-REM sleep. The EEG may show focal or multifocal slow spike-waves predominantly in centro-temporal, frontal, and less frequently, parieto-occipital regions similar to those observed in idiopathic epilepsy of childhood (*figure 1*). Fast spikes, polyspikes, asymmetries, and paroxysmal voltage attenuations, evocative of forms of structural epilepsies, as well as

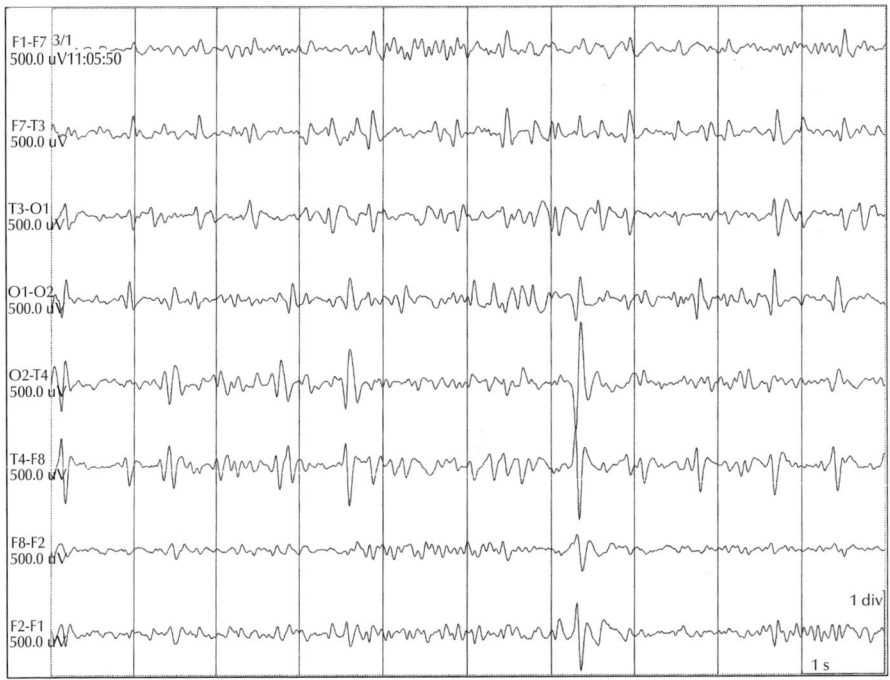

Figure 1/ A five-year-old boy who had a focal motor seizure during sleep. The EEG recording during sleep shows independent bilateral spikes.

diffuse spike-wave paroxysms at 2.5-3 Hz, may be seen (Caraballo et al., 2013a). After the initial period in which the interictal EEG shows focal abnormalities, the appearance of some particular EEG manifestations, such as an increase of focal abnormalities during sleep and while awake, and bilateral spikes and waves predominantly in the anterior region that increase during sleep may suggest a probable evolution to the CSWS period (*figure 2*).

In the second stage, the seizures become more frequent and complicated with typical or, more frequently, atypical absences, myoclonic absences, absence status epilepticus, atonic or clonic seizures, and generalized tonic-clonic seizures. Tonic seizures do not occur. In this period, the mean age at epilepsy onset is 6.8 years (range: 4-13 years). The interictal activity is much more frequent and severe with more widespread spikes of higher amplitude associated with a more abnormal background. During sleep, the EEG pattern shows CSWS (*figure 3*). The onset of CSWS is accompanied by psychomotor decline with deterioration of IQ, language (expressive aphasia and articulation disorder as well as auditory verbal agnosia), cognitive functions, and behavior (hyperkinesis and bizarre, aggressive, psychotic or autistic behavior, emotional instability) (Seri et al., 2009; Seegmuller et al., 2012). Motor impairment, such as pseudoataxia and even loss of independent gait, worsening of a unilateral deficit, fine motor clumsiness with distorted handwriting, dyspraxia, and dystonia have been described (Fejerman et al., 2000; Seegmuller et al., 2012). In a historical series of 209 published patients with CSWS, Rousselle and Revol (1995) recognized three clinical groups based on neuropsychological profile during the CSWS period. This profile correlated directly with the duration of CSWS and the site of the main epileptogenic focus: Group 1 showed no neuropsychological deterioration. In these children the period of CSWS was of shorter duration and the main epileptiform focus had a Rolandic topography.

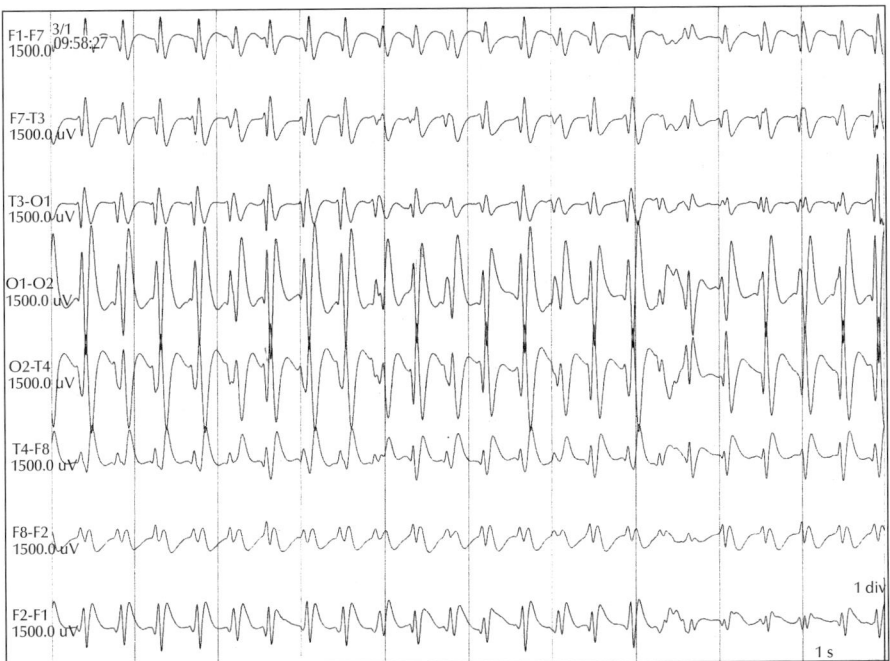

Figure 2/ The EEG recording during sleep shows high-frequency spikes in frontal regions.

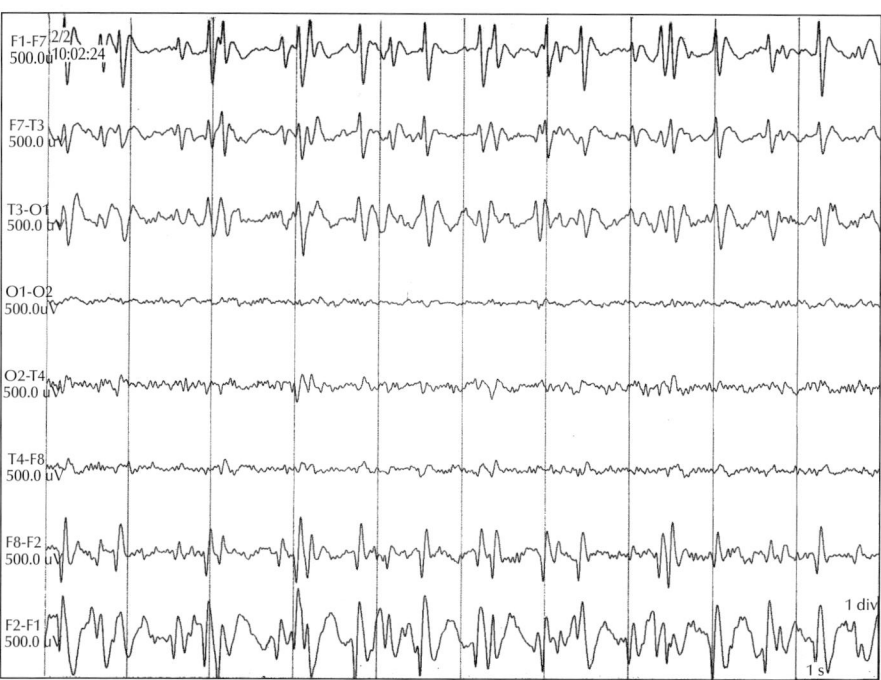

Figure 3/ An eight-year-old boy with negative myoclonia, motor deterioraton, and behavioral disturbances associated with right posterior polymicrogyria. The EEG recording during sleep shows continuous spikes and waves during slow sleep predominantly in the right occipital region.

In Group 2, children had language deterioration (primarily LKS) and the main epileptiform focus found was in the temporal region. In Group 3 (the largest group), children had global neuropsychological deterioration rather than linguistic impairment. The main epileptiform focus was found in the frontal region. Recently, we have reported a series of patients with focal CSWS. Those with focal CSWS in the frontal region showed behavioral disturbances and/or motor deterioration and in those with temporo-occipital involvement language and/or behavioral disturbances were seen (Caraballo et al., 2015). In another study, two patients with acquired Kanji dysgraphia who developed CSWS that was dominant in the occipito-temporal region were described showing morphological, phonemic, and semantic errors (Kuki et al., 2014). Focal CSWS is an intriguing and challenging entity and this finding underlines the importance of an adequate neurophysiological examination, to localize the functional lesion, as well as a thorough neuropsychological evaluation in individual cases to understand the impact of these particular EEG findings during sleep on brain function (Tassinari et al., 2015).

In the third stage (after months to usually two to seven years), the seizures remit and a general improvement can be seen. Whether or not EEG abnormalities persist after the CSWS has disappeared depends on the underlying etiology. Therefore, the interictal sleep and awake EEG should normalize in idiopathic or probably genetic cases. In structural cases, the EEG recordings may show focal, multifocal, or bilateral asymmetric spikes (Caraballo et al., 2013a). After the CSWS has disappeared, school performances and IQ may improve significantly in seizure-free patients and in those who have a more than 75% seizure reduction

(Caraballo et al., 2013a). A recent study has suggested a correlation between neuropsychological outcome and recovery of physiological sleep homeostasis, as measured by impairment of sleep slow-wave activity (SSWA) during ESES and SSWA renormalization after CSWS resolution (Bolsterli et al., Epilepsia, 2017; see also Rubboli et al., p. 69-76).

In children with structural or idiopathic focal epilepsies, classic antiepileptic drugs, such as carbamazepine, oxcarbazepine, phenobarbital, or phenytoin, may induce the appearance of CSWS; these should be avoided (Fejerman et al., 2000). Similar effects have been reported in sporadic cases with valproic acid, lamotrigine, topiramate, and levetiracetam; these findings await further confirmation (Fejerman et al., 2000). To our knowledge, this phenomenon has not been observed in patients using clobazam, ethosuximide, and sulthiame.

■ Outcome and prognosis

Seizures almost always disappear with age, even in patients with a static or progressive encephalopathy (Bureau, 1995; Guerrini et al., 1998; Tassinari et al., 2000; Loddenkemper et al., 2011; Caraballo et al., 2013a; Sánchez Fernández et al., 2013). Thus, this pattern is independent of the etiological lesion, as shown by the age-related remission, also in patients with a malformation of cortical development or a progressive neurodegenerative disease (Loddenkemper et al., 2011). Seizure freedom has been reported at around 6-9 years of age, but data are scarce (Sánchez Fernández et al., 2013). In any case, clinical seizures tend to remit spontaneously around puberty. The mean duration of epilepsy is 12 years (range: 4-15 years). CSWS also disappears in all cases, with an average persistence until 11 years of age (Tassinari et al., 2000). Focal abnormalities instead, may persist for some time after the disappearance of CSWS (Bureau, 1995). The disappearance of the clinical seizures and CSWS may be simultaneous or seizures may disappear before or after disappearance of the CSWS pattern on the EEG (Bureau, 1995).

Electroclinical parameters in the pre-CSWS period that have been proposed to predict a poor outcome are early-onset seizures, appearance of new seizures, a significant increase in seizure frequency, and resistance to a single AED (Dalla Bernardina et al., 1989; Kramer et al., 2009; Seri et al., 2009). From the electrical point of view, an increase in the frequency of the interictal EEG paroxysms while awake and during sleep, bilateral spike-and-wave paroxysms predominantly in anterior regions, and frequent generalized paroxysms may also be predictive of a poor evolution in CSWS (Dalla Bernardina et al., 1989).

When CSWS disappears, neurocognitive and behavioral status improve, but residual moderate to severe neurocognitive impairments might persist (see also Arzimanoglou and Cross, p. 77-81). Cognitive deterioration remains unchanged in almost one third of the patients, the majority of whom are structural cases.

In our study of 117 patients with the CSWS syndrome (Caraballo et al., 2013a), around 70% of the structural and idiopathic cases regained their previous cognitive level. Similar findings were published in earlier reports (Liukkonen et al., 2010).

A study on the long-term outcome after cognitive and behavioral regression in non-lesional epilepsy with CSWS revealed that cognitive recovery after cessation of the CSWS depends on the severity and duration of the initial regression (Saltik et al., 2005).

The duration of the CSWS seems to be the most important predictor of cognitive outcome (Bureau, 1995; De Negri, 1997). Early recognition and effective therapy to reduce the seizures and resolve the CSWS may be crucial to improve long-term prognosis (Inutsuka et al., 2006). Cognitive recovery is observed in patients that respond well to AED treatment, and further deterioration is halted in the symptomatic/structural and non-idiopathic group. In patients who do not respond to AEDs, however, cognition continues to deteriorate (Caraballo et al., 2013a).

In our study (Caraballo et al., 2013a), outcome depended on the etiology. The idiopathic group had an excellent prognosis. In the symptomatic/structural and non-idiopathic group, the patients with unilateral polymicrogyria had a relatively good prognosis compared to children with other structural etiologies. Typical EEG findings before and during the CSWS period, such as asymmetric background activity, focal fast spikes, slow waves, polyspikes, and paroxysmal voltage attenuation, were only seen in the symptomatic/structural and non-idiopathic group.

Fejerman et al. found that children with an atypical evolution of BCECTS evolving into ABPEC and SEBCECTS had an ultimate good prognosis, while cases evolving into LKS and ECSWS syndrome had a guarded prognosis in terms of language or cognitive and behavioral impairments (Fejerman et al., 2000). The outcome of Landau-Kleffner syndrome is variable, however, the prognosis is usually better than that of CSWS (Van Hirtum-Das et al., 2006). The seizures generally respond well to antiepileptic drugs and EEG abnormalities disappear after a few years (Caraballo et al., 2014). The language disorder, however, may never resolve in almost half of the patients (Soprano et al., 1994). As in patients with a structural etiology, the prognosis is often not benign. Early recognition and adequate treatment management may avoid cognitive deterioration and surgical intervention (Caraballo et al., 2013b).

■ Conclusions

The CSWS syndrome is a well-defined disorder associated with focal or apparently generalized seizures, a peculiar EEG pattern, motor impairment, and cognitive deterioration. Both seizures and CSWS disappear over time in the majority of patients. Neuropsychological outcome is often poor. Although CSWS disappears around puberty, epilepsy and cognitive outcome depend on etiology. The age at onset of CSWS and the site of the main epileptogenic focus may influence long-term neuropsychological outcome and CSWS duration may affect severity of neuropsychological involvement. Cognitive recovery occurs in children who respond to antiepileptic drugs while it continues to deteriorate in those who do not. Further deterioration is halted in the structural group.

EEG features in Encephalopathy related to Status Epilepticus during slow Sleep

Elena Gardella, Gaetano Cantalupo, Pål G. Larsson,
Elena Fontana, Bernardo dalla Bernardina, Guido Rubboli,
Francesca Darra

Since the first description in 1971 (Patry *et al.*), the peculiar EEG pattern during sleep of ESES represents, by definition, one of the main features and at the same time a key element for its diagnosis. The alternative term "Continuous Spikes and Waves during slow Sleep" (CSWS), accepted in 1989 also by the Commission on Classification and Terminology of the International League against Epilepsy (ILAE) further emphasizes the EEG picture as a cardinal element of this syndrome.

Even if the first "E" in the acronym "ESES" was initially meant to indicate "Electrical" SES (Patry *et al.*, 1971), a few years later Tassinari and colleagues (1977) suggested the use of "E" for "Encephalopathy" with SES after noting that "the condition of a protracted SES can be the factor leading to severe mental deterioration and psychic disturbances". This early communication introduced *in nuce* the concept of Epileptic Encephalopathy, later on proposed by the International League Against Epilepsy (ILAE) Classification Task Force (1989).

Currently, ESES is defined as an age-related and self-limiting disorder (Tassinari *et al*, 2019; ILAE Commission, 1989), characterized by:

- a typical EEG pattern, consisting of a striking exaggeration of epileptic discharges during NREM sleep for a protracted period of time (months or years);
- a clinical picture based on global or selective cognitive regression/stagnation, behavioral disorders, motor deficits, with or without overt epileptic seizures.

■ EEG features

The most typical and easily recognizable pattern of ESES consists of the sudden appearance at drowsiness of (sub-)continuous diffuse epileptic activity represented by synchronous and rhythmic high-amplitude spikes and waves (SW), persisting during all NREM-sleep stages (*figure 1A*). In this condition, the sleep physiological graphoelements, particularly sleep spindles, can be difficult to detect. The SW may become slower and more rhythmic during slow sleep (*figure 1B*), sometimes producing a fragmented EEG pattern (Veggiotti *et al.*, 2001) (*figure 2*).

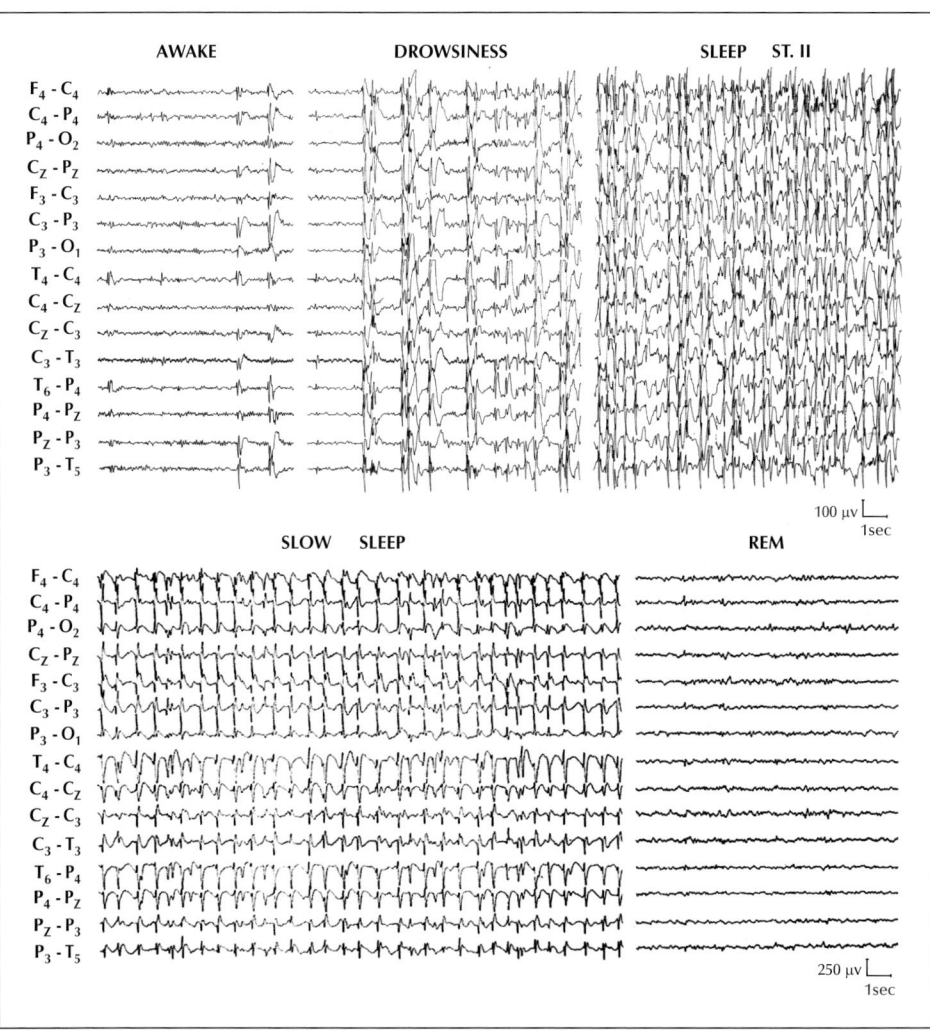

Figure 1/ Male, 11 years and three months old. (A) Upper panel. The EEG during wakefulness is characterized by spike-and-waves in the right and left centro-parietal regions, with sudden exaggeration and diffuse spreading during drowsiness. During NREM Stage 2 sleep, the EEG shows continuous, diffuse and rhythmic spikes and waves with high amplitude. (B) Lower panel. The spike-and-waves become slower and more rhythmic during slow sleep and more focal during REM sleep, resembling the EEG activity during wakefulness.

Focal epileptiform abnormalities during wakefulness can be inconstantly seen also during sleep as focal spikes intermixed with the diffuse SW. In some cases, a focal slow activity is also present, reflecting the localization of the main epileptic focus, and probably contributing to the symptoms as well (Massa et al., 2000; Tassinari et al., 2000; Aeby et al., 2005; Dalla Bernardina et al., 2005) (figure 3).

During REM sleep, the diffuse discharges are replaced by more focal SW, resembling those observed during wakefulness (figure 1). Sometimes, brief bursts of diffuse SW can appear also during REM sleep, but this is usually in concomitance with an arousal.

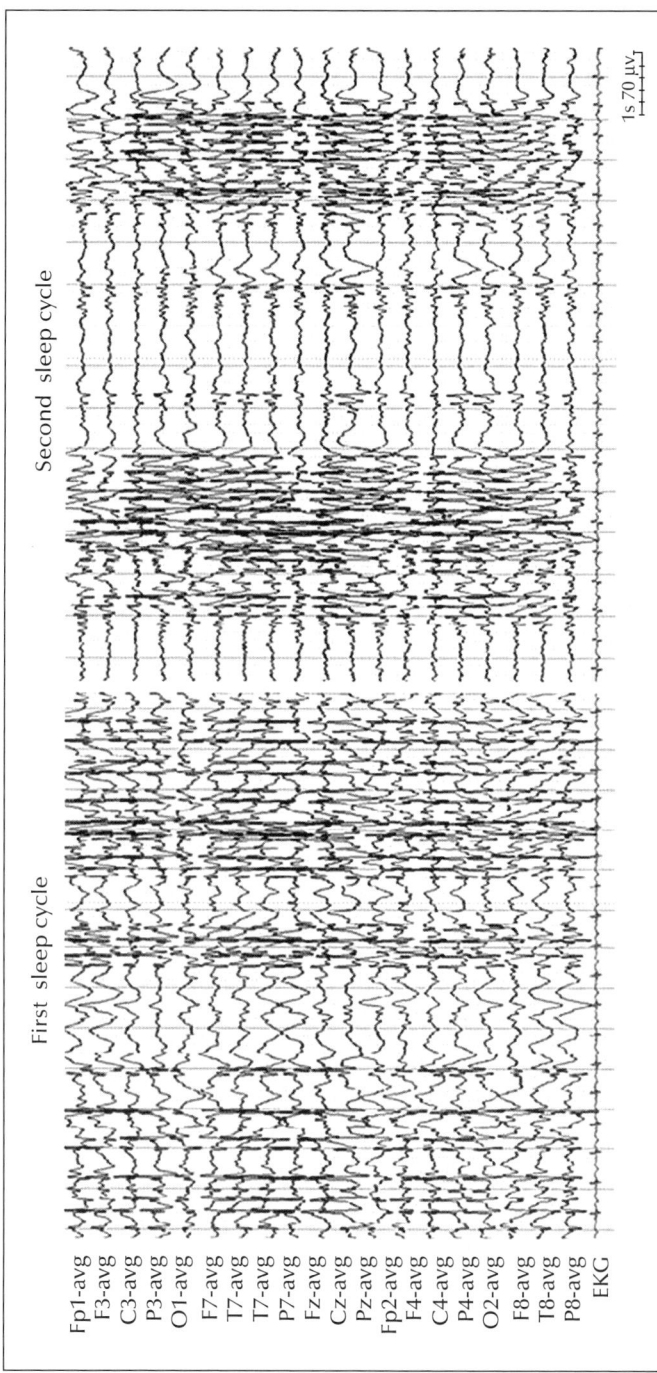

Figure 2/ Fluctuations of EEG pattern during the night. Male, 11 years old. Symptomatic ESES on therapy with levetiracetam, valproic acid, and baclofen. The SW distribution changes from a continuous pattern during the first cycle of sleep (left panel) to a more fragmented pattern during the second sleep cycle (right panel). The global SWI during NREM sleep was 83%.

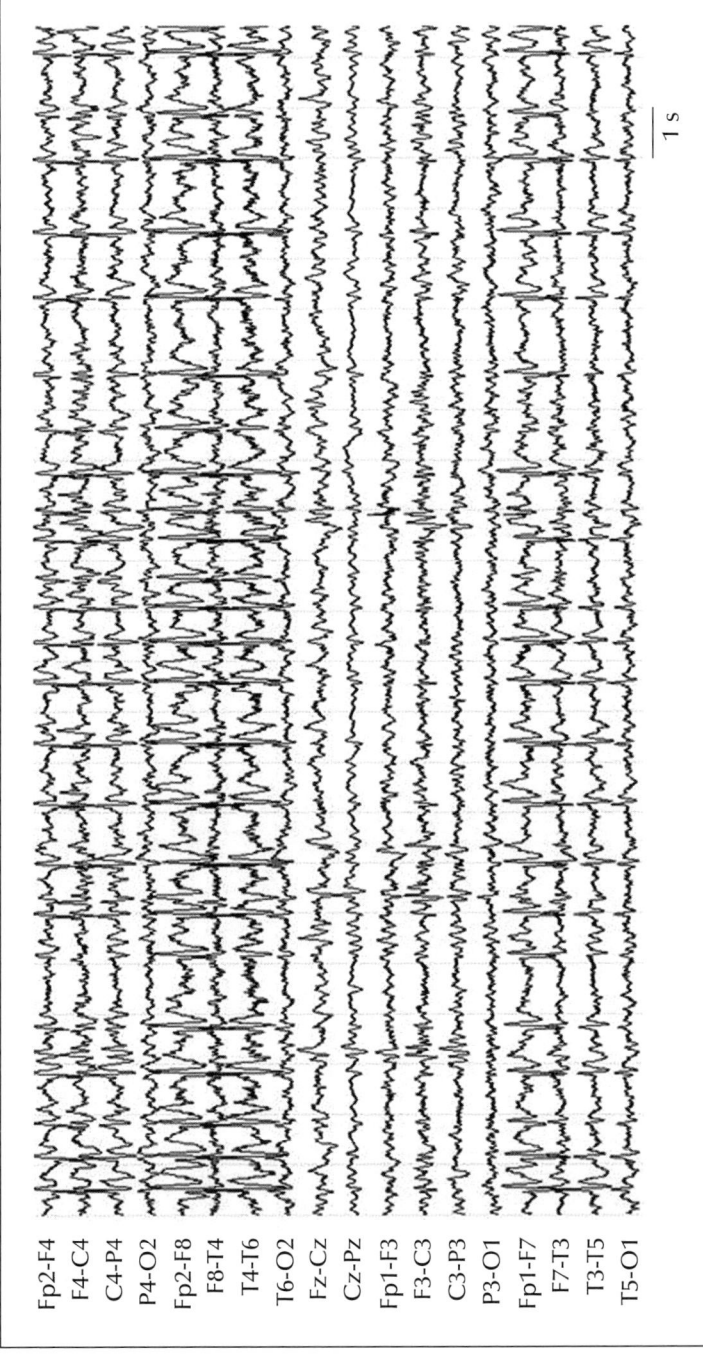

Figure 3/ Focal slow components and "false multifocality". Female, eight years old, with idiopathic ESES. Subcontinuous rhythmical SW in the right centro-temporal regions rapidly spreading to homologous regions of the contralateral hemisphere (producing a bilateral focal status); the leading hemisphere is the right, in which we observe a predominance in amplitude, a constant anticipation of the right discharges over the left ones, and continuous delta activity interomingled with SW.

The continuous and diffuse EEG pattern during NREM sleep results from a secondary bilateral synchronization of the focal/multifocal SW observed during wakefulness (*figure 1*). In other cases, the spreading of the discharges is unilateral, leading to a hemispheric ESES (Hirsch *et al.*, 1995; Galanopoulou *et al.*, 2000) (*figure 4*).

In some patients, the ESES pattern can be strictly focal (*figure 5A*) (Aeby *et al.*, 2005; Tassinari *et al.*, 2019; Caraballo *et al.*, 2015) or unilateral, eventually spreading to the

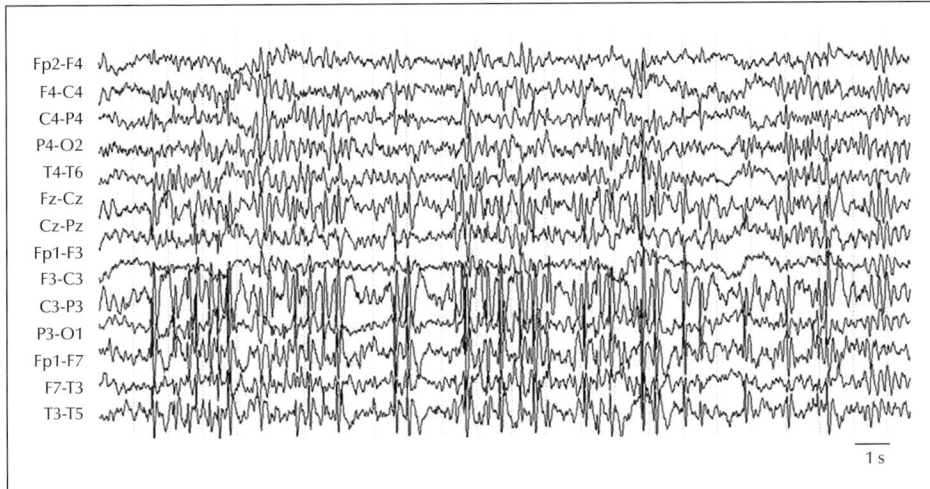

Figure 4/ Hemispheric ESES (Hemi-ESES). Female, three years old. Cryptogenic ESES with epileptiform abnormalities involving the entire left hemisphere with occasional spreading to a Rolandic area of the right hemisphere.

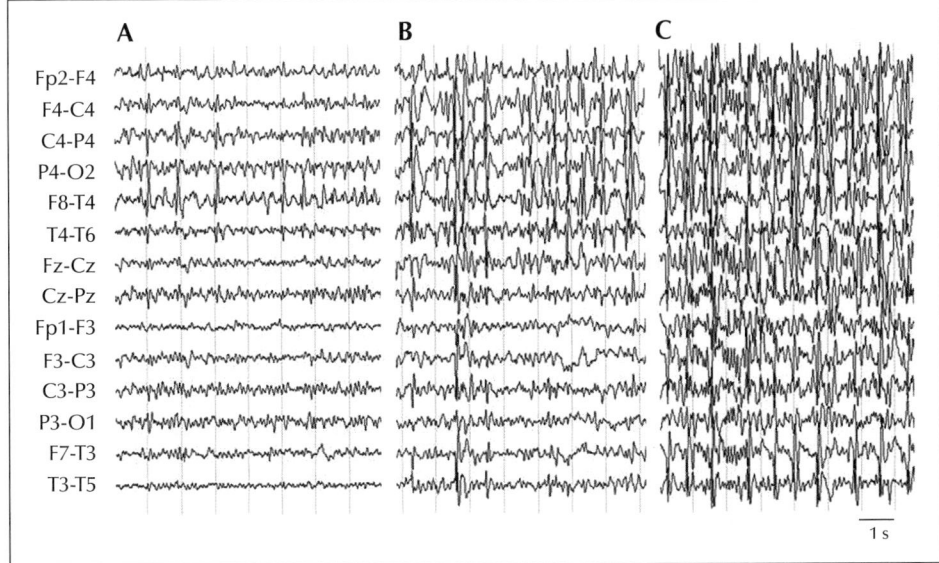

Figure 5/ EEG topography evolution during the ESES course in the same patient. Three different sleep recordings in the same little girl with symptomatic ESES due to a right parietal polymicrogyria. The EEG pattern changes from focal (A: age six years, eight months) to hemispheric (B: age six years, 11 months) and diffuse (C: age seven years).

homologous contralateral regions, giving the false impression of multi-focality (*figure 3*). A bilateral ESES EEG pattern can result from a striking activation of focal paroxysms, independently on the two hemispheres. Often multifocal paroxysms show an independent and alternating increase in frequency on the two hemispheres. In these focal/multifocal cases, the spike frequency can be relatively high during REM sleep as well. Moreover, the activation of multiple independent foci can vary in the different stages of sleep. In cases of multiple foci, it might be relevant to compute the contribution of each single focus to the total spike-wave-index (SWI) separately (*figure 6*) (see also Peltola *et al.*, 2014), which is the percentage of time occupied by SW discharges (Patry *et al.*, 1971; see also below).

The unilateral, focal or multifocal ESES patterns can be interpreted as the result of an abnormal activation of SW abnormalities during NREM sleep, without secondary bilateral synchronization (which can appear eventually, later on, during ESES evolution). An early recognition of these patterns at ESES onset might help to clarify whether they have different etiological, physio-pathological and prognostic significance. During ESES evolution, a transition between diffuse, hemispheric and focal patterns can be observed in a given patient, possibly depending on the spontaneous fluctuations of the disease and on the ongoing therapy (*figure 5*) (Gordon, 2000; Holmes and Lenck-Santini, 2006).

Often, the introduction of a medical treatment tends to render the EEG pattern more focal (*figure 7*), however, the opposite is also possible (for instance, with carbamazepine and oxcarbazepine) (Dalla Bernardina *et al.*, 2005; Pavlidis *et al.*, 2015).

The morphology and amplitude of the epileptiform activity has been infrequently reported as a relevant parameter. In most patients, the epileptiform abnormalities during ESES are an exaggeration of the epileptiform activities before ESES onset, and their morphology ultimately depends on the epilepsy type. Consequently, the analysis of the morphology of the EEG abnormalities during both wakefulness and sleep might be a valuable parameter for a syndromic and/or etiological assessment of ESES (Dalla Bernardina *et al.*, 2005).

The *topography of the epileptiform activity* can be extremely variable among different patients with ESES, in the same patients at different recordings, and even at different times during the same EEG recording.

The EEG of patients with epilepsy before ESES onset can show focal or multifocal epileptiform abnormalities, with the primary focus in the fronto-central, centro-temporal, temporal, parietal, occipital regions as well as in the vertex, depending on the type of epilepsy syndrome. Independent of the pre-ESES EEG topography, an EEG feature that can indicate evolution into ESES is the migration of the SW bilaterally to the frontal regions, moving back to their original topography at the time of ESES offset (either spontaneous or due to treatment) (Dalla Bernardina *et al.*, 1978, 1984, 1989, 2005).

Therefore, the topography as well as the sleep-wake distribution of the epileptiform abnormalities during the evolution of ESES can vary significantly. In addition, the characteristics of the EEG pattern can be also influenced by the developmental stage and, as already mentioned, by ongoing therapy. Finally, some authors emphasize the importance of the localization and orientation of the spike-related EEG dipoles in the definition of the EEG pattern (Morrell *et al.*, 1995; Galanopoulou *et al.*, 2000).

At variance with the diagnostic importance of a high SWI during NREM sleep in ESES, relatively little attention has been paid to the features and clinical correlation of the EEG

EEG features in Encephalopathy related to Status Epilepticus during slow Sleep

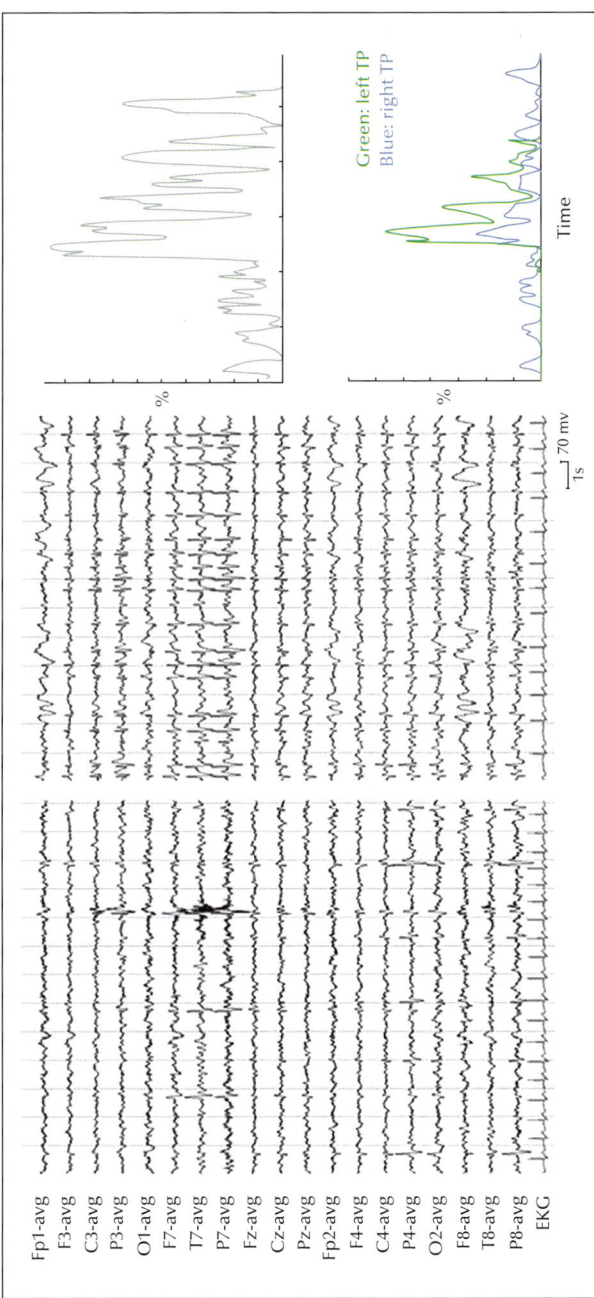

Figure 6/ Two independent foci. A girl, eleven years and seven months old, affected by early developmental dysphasia; she had never had seizures. The ongoing therapy was sulthiame 250 mg/die. The EEG during wakefulness shows two independent foci in the right and left rolandic regions. Note the change in side prevalence from wakefulness (right parieto-occipital regions; left panel) to NREM sleep (left temporo-parietal regions; middle panel). Right panels: The SWI during NREM sleep is 66% (max. activation 96%). The NREM sleep/wakefulness SWI ratio is 5.9. The upper panel shows the fluctuations of the cumulative SWI (both foci) during the 24-hour EEG and the lower panel shows the SWI for each single focus, showing a prevalent activation of the right epileptic focus during wakefulness and a significant predominant activation of the left focus (the side of speech dominance) during NREM sleep.

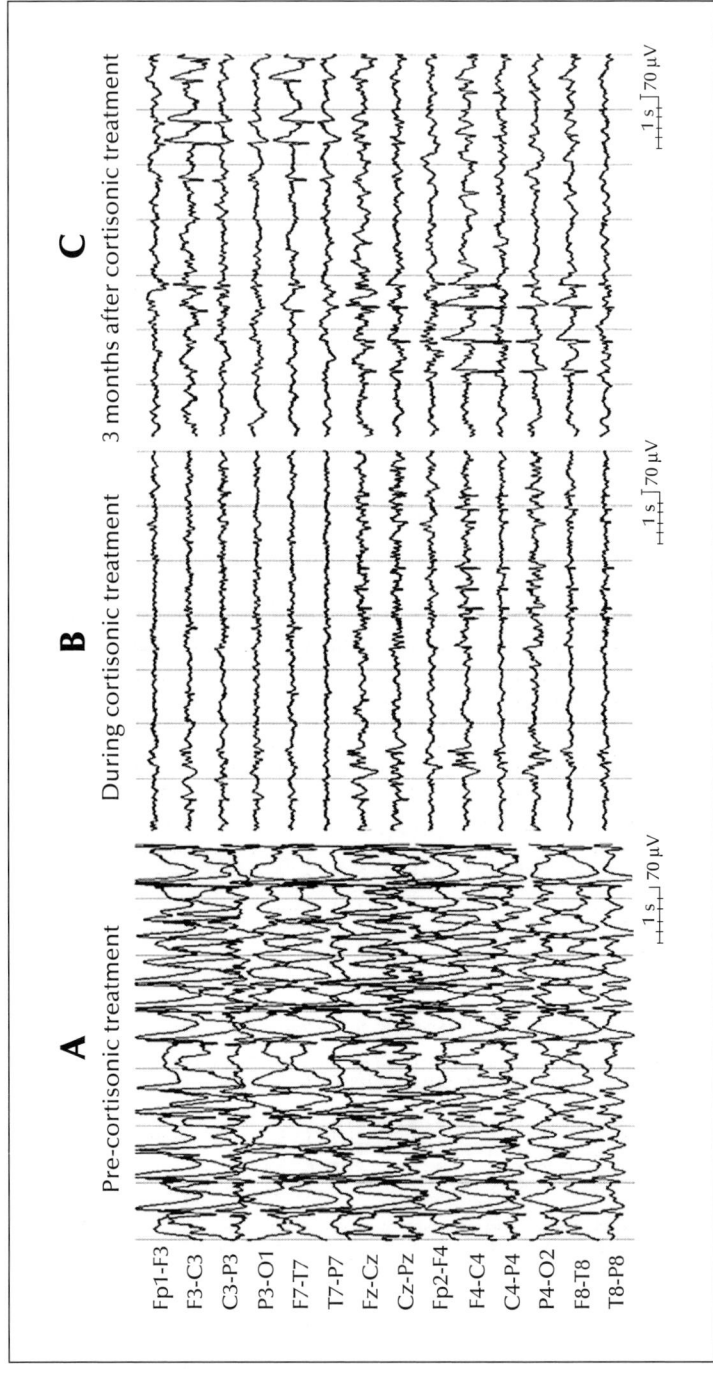

Figure 7/ Effects of medical treatment. A nine-year-old boy with atypical benign partial epilepsy evolving to ESES and ADHD. In July 2010 (A), the patient's clinical picture worsened, (B) during steroid therapy - for 4 weeks with gradual withdrawal until November 2010. On February 2011 (C), the patient's condition was stable. The good clinical as well as EEG effects of steroid therapy partially continued.

epileptic activity *during wakefulness*. Actually, this aspect can bear diagnostic and prognostic relevance (Dalla Bernardina et al., 1989). In patients with a typical ESES pattern during sleep, the EEG activity during wakefulness can consist of: (a) fairly focal SW (*figure 1*); (b) a frequent burst of diffuse SW, often with impairment of consciousness (atypical absences); (c) diffuse SW, often associated with absences with negative motor (atonic) or myoclonic component (*figure 8*). In these latter cases, the abrupt appearance of seizures during wakefulness can allow a timely diagnosis and a prompt therapeutic intervention (Dalla Bernardina et al., 1989). However, in some cases the medical treatment can significantly improve the EEG picture during wakefulness, without modifying the ESES pattern. Therefore, even in the case of a dramatic EEG improvement during wakefulness, a sleep EEG should be performed.

The organization of the EEG background is also a relevant parameter. Sleep/wake architecture, as well as the sleep macrostructure are usually well preserved during ESES (Hirsch et al., 1995), whereas, sleep microstructure (Nobili et al., 2001) and slow wave activity during sleep (Bölsterli et al., 2011; 2017) may be impaired.

■ Measures in ESES

EEG recording techniques in ESES

Various approaches have been adopted to record the EEG epileptiform activity related to ESES, ranging from a 24-hour EEG, sleep EEG (whole night or afternoon sleep) or polysomnography with or without video registration and with or without sleep medication (for a review, see Scheltens-de Boer, 2009).

The first NREM sleep cycle is a period of particular activation of epileptiform abnormalities; usually this activation decreases in the subsequent nocturnal sleep cycles. Therefore, an afternoon sleep EEG, including wakefulness and drowsiness, may be sufficient as a first screening, but for a correct diagnosis a full-night EEG recording is recommended (Gardella et al., 2016).

The *percentage of epileptiform activity during sleep* can be expressed as SWI, defined as the percentage of NREM sleep occupied by spikes and waves (Tassinari et al., 2000; see also Cantalupo et al., p. 37-48). Different cut-off values have been adopted, ranging from 85% to 90% (Tassinari et al., 2000) to 25% (Van Hirtum-Das et al., 2006). These inconsistencies depend mainly on the lack of accepted criteria for the diagnosis of ESES. Moreover, as mentioned before, the different methodologies that have been used to measure the SWI and the evidence of SWI fluctuations in the same patient during the course of ESES may have further hampered the identification of a shared SWI threshold, and how and when it should be assessed. Even though it is quite exceptional that a SWI ≥80% is not associated with any cognitive, behavioral and/or motor disorder, the diagnosis of ESES cannot be based only on the measurement of the SWI. Indeed, ESES can be diagnosed only when there is evidence of an appearance or worsening of a neuropsychological impairment, associated with a striking increase of the epileptic activity during sleep.

Quantitative variation of the epileptiform activity during the night is sporadically mentioned (Tassinari et al., 2000; Galanopoulou et al., 2000; Larsson et al., 2010), most often reporting an increase of the epileptic activity during the first part of the night. An accentuation of the epileptic discharges can be observed in the period preceding the sleep onset (*figure 9*). Some

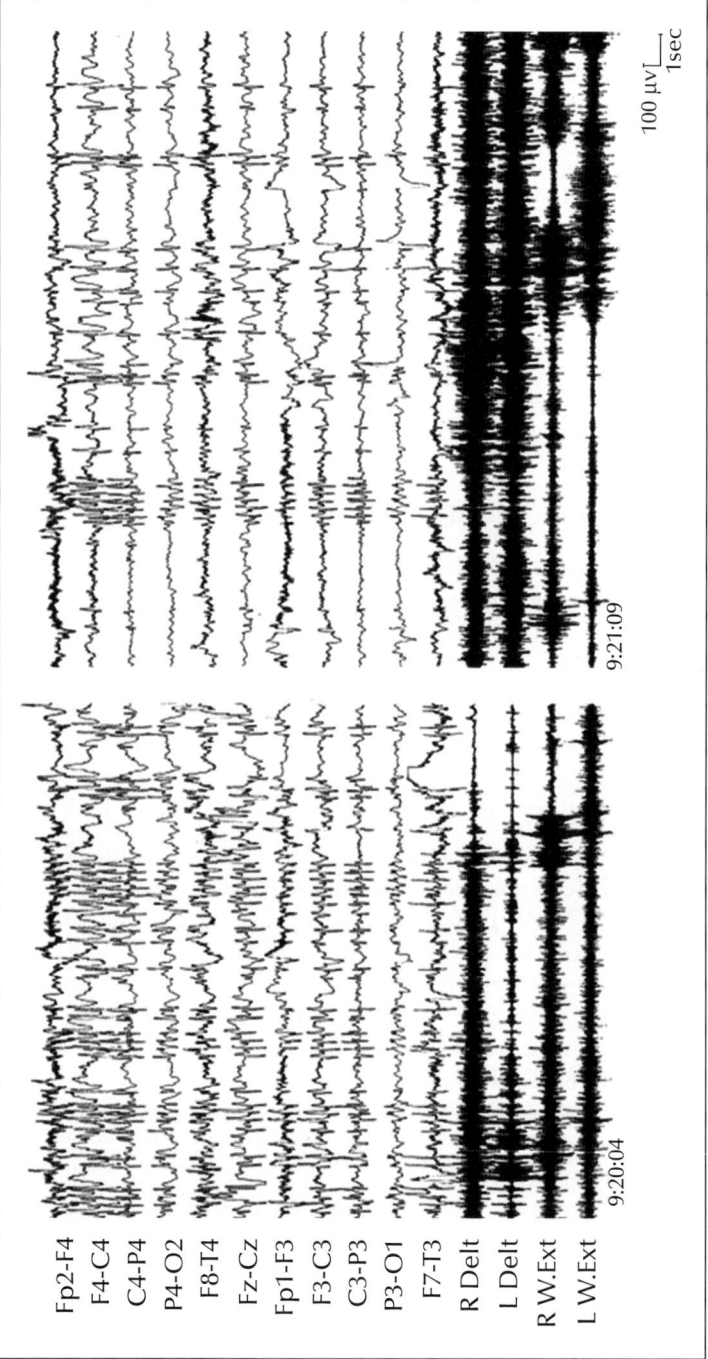

Figure 8/ EEG and clinical features during wakefulness. A child, three years and five months old, with ESES. The EEG during wakefulness shows trains of irregular SW complexes, associated with atypical absences with myoclonic and atonic phenomena.

EEG features in Encephalopathy related to Status Epilepticus during slow Sleep

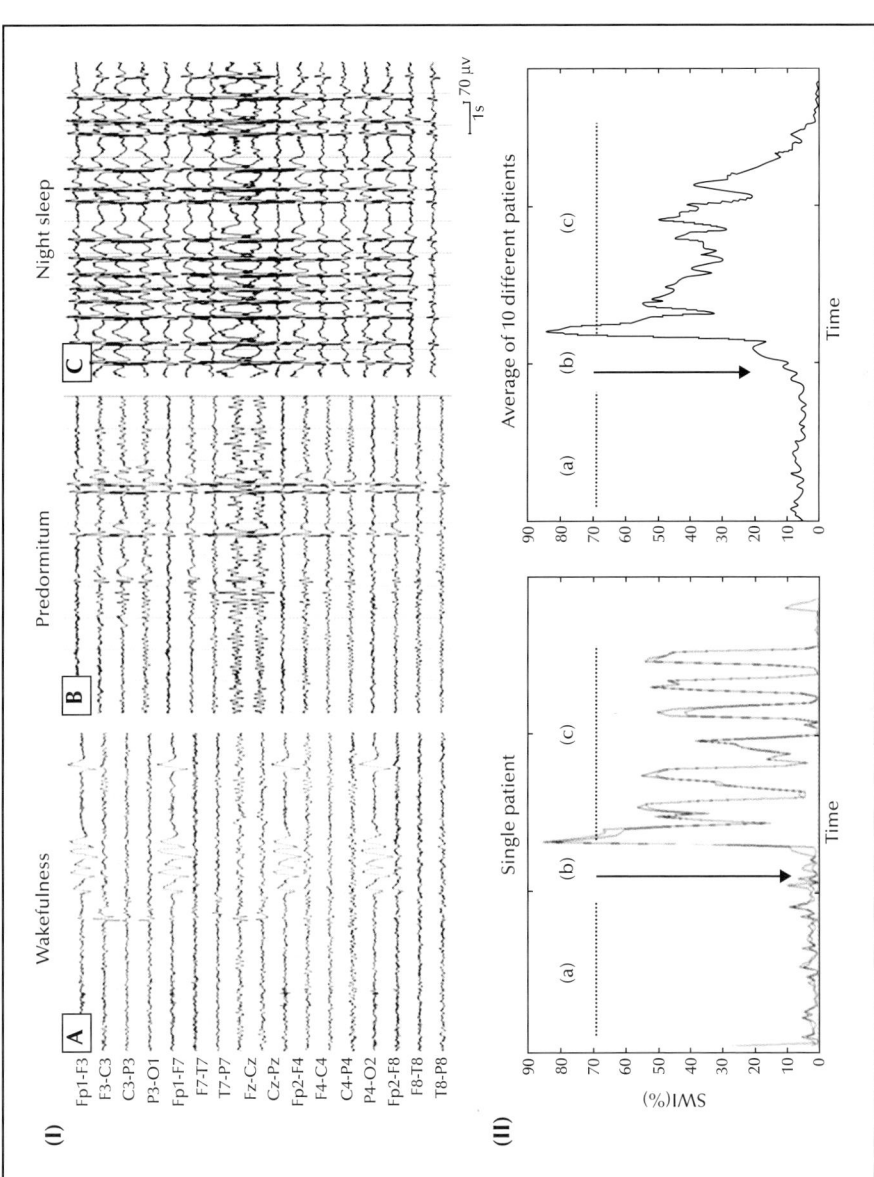

Figure 9/ Distribution of epileptiform abnormalities during a 24-hour EEG. Lower panels: fluctuation of the SWI during the 24-hour EEG recordings in a single patient (left) - shown in *Figure 1* - and fluctuation of average SWI of 10 different patients (right). For the computation of the SWI average, the EEG recordings of the 10 patients have been aligned to the onset of the nocturnal sleep. The graphs show low values of SWI during wakefulness (A), gradual, slight increase of the SWI in the period preceding the night sleep (B), and a sudden increase of the SWI at sleep onset, persisting during NREM night sleep, and decreasing during the REM phases, reflecting the physiological sleep macrostructure.

data have also shown that the computation of the SWI during a short sleep period, *e.g.* an afternoon EEG, might be in some cases misleading with a lower diagnostic yield as compared to overnight EEG recording (Gardella *et al.*, 2016; Cantalupo *et al.*, p. 37-48).

▪ Some clinical considerations

ESES can occur as a single episode of variable duration and can recur as several episodes with more or less prolonged intervals. During follow-up, during the course of ESES, the epileptic discharges in sleep tend to become more focal and the SWI tend to decrease. In addition, in the active phase of ESES, fluctuations in the clinical picture (cognitive/behavioral impairment or seizure frequency) may not be paralleled by changes of the EEG features (such as SWI, topography, morphology, amplitude and sleep-wakefulness distribution of the discharges) (Morikawa *et al.*, 1985; Hommet *et al.*, 2000; Sánchez Fernández *et al.*, 2012). For these reasons, the diagnosis and the monitoring of ESES requires both repeated EEG and neuropsychological investigations.

Receptive aphasia has been shown to be related to epileptic activity during sleep in the temporal regions, whereas a global cognitive decline with behavioral problems has been associated with frontal or diffuse spike topography (Beaumanoir, 1995; Tassinari *et al.*, 2000). Therefore, the neuropsychological assessment should also take into account the topography of the EEG epileptic discharges, in particular in those cases with focal ESES that might cause very selective cognitive deficits (Kuki *et al.*, 2015).

Additional parameters such as overt or subclinical seizure frequency, the age at ESES onset, and ESES duration could also be involved and require further studies to investigate their possible role in determining the ESES clinical features.

▪ Conclusions

ESES is a peculiar electro-clinical entity whose main EEG characteristic is an extreme activation of paroxysmal activity during sleep, probably subtended by an age-dependent mechanism. Secondary bilateral synchrony contributes to the spread of focal epileptic discharges during sleep. The main EEG parameter, that has been assessed since the first description of ESES, is the SWI. However, establishing a minimum SWI for the diagnosis of ESES is somewhat arbitrary, mainly because of the lack of shared criteria and because of the diversity of measurement methods used in the different studies. Additional aspects that have to be taken into account in the evaluation of the EEG during ESES are the heterogeneity of the EEG features (such as, for instance, topography of the epileptic abnormalities and pattern of spread) that may change in a given patient at different time points of the disease course, but sometimes even in the same recording, and/or may depend on the ongoing therapy. On the other hand, it must be emphasized that the diagnosis of ESES cannot rely solely on the assessment of the SWI and/or other EEG features but requires demonstration of a neuropsychological/behavioral derangement associated with the appearance of the peculiar sleep EEG pattern.

▪ Acknowledgements

This research was supported by the European Union Seventh Framework Program FP7 under the project DESIRE (grant agreement 602531) to GC, BDB and FD.

Quantitative EEG analysis in Encephalopathy related to Status Epilepticus during slow Sleep

Gaetano Cantalupo, Elena Pavlidis, Sandor Beniczky, Pietro Avanzini, Elena Gardella, Pål G. Larsson

The quantitative analysis of EEG plays a fundamental role in the diagnosis of Encephalopathy related to Status Epilepticus during slow Sleep (ESES). In fact, since its first description (Patry et al., 1971), a computable measure of epileptiform discharge (ED) abundance during sleep was used as a diagnostic criterion. Along the lines of Tassinari's hypothesis - that the severity of encephalopathy is proportional to the amount of sleep substituted by spike-and-wave complexes - the description of the EEG pattern of ESES has been based almost exclusively on the abundance of EDs, while other quantitative and qualitative measures have been usually neglected (Scheltens-de Boer, 2009; Tassinari et al., 2019; Peltola et al., 2014). However, nowadays it is becoming increasingly clear that this variable alone does not explain the whole clinical course of the patients. The aim of this paper was not to merely illustrate the best quantitative measure, but rather to provide the reader with a number of quantitative variables potentially useful to reach a reliable electro-clinical correlation. These quantitative measures can be related to the amount and quality of epileptiform paroxysmal activities but also to physiological components of sleep. Furthermore, we will examine the possible pitfalls and discrepancies in the methods currently used in the ESES/CSWS literature.

■ Epileptiform activities

Amount

Spike-and-wave index(es)

In the 70s, at the Centre Saint-Paul in Marseille, the quantification of EDs in ESES was inspired by the recently adopted (at that time) Rechtschaffen and Kales (1968) sleep scoring method (Tassinari personal communication), in which, for each epoch, the time occupied by an activity (e.g. delta waves) is expressed as percentage and serves as a scoring criterion. Accordingly, the amount of EDs was expressed as the percentage of the total duration of slow sleep occupied by a spike and the following slow wave or by sequences of rhythmic spike-and-wave complexes. This percentage was referred as "spike and wave index" (SWI) in the seminal paper by Patry et al. (1971), in which six patients were selected based on the "spectacular increase" of the spike-and-waves observed as soon as they fell asleep. In this selected population, the SI ranged from 85 to 100% and these values were used as a reference for the typical feature of overnight EEG in patients with ESES. The method of determining SI was not described in the paper, and as a consequence, a number of different methods were crafted and used to determine the SWI.

The great majority of the subsequent studies continued to rely on visual estimation, without further clarifying the computational rules to determine the percentage of time occupied by the pathologic pattern, with the exception of the study by Aeby et al. (2005), in which it is specified that the SWI was obtained by calculating the percentage of 1-second bins containing at least one spike-and-wave complex (Aeby et al., 2005). This method is similar to the "original" since even a one-second interval between two spike-and-wave complexes is computed as discharge-free. However, only 60 minutes of EEG were analyzed instead of the full night.

The introduction of digital EEG systems offered an opportunity to reduce the workload needed for SWI assessment of the entire nocturnal recording. In fact, a number of computer-aided spike detection methods have been developed and some of these successfully applied to ESES/CSWS (Larsson et al., 2009; Nonclerq et al., 2009; Nonclerq et al., 2012; Peltola et al., 2012; Scherg et al., 2012; Chavakula et al., 2013; Joshi et al., 2018). A spike-detection algorithm is used to find each spike (with or without an aftercoming slow-wave) within the EEG (with different sensitivity and specificity based on the method used). These time points can be used to calculate the discharge-free interval, based on the assumption that a minimum interval between consecutive spikes (Inter-Spike Interval - ISI) is required to consider it as discharge-free. The first to use this approach to determine SWI in ESES were Larsson and coworkers (2009), documenting that ISI equal to 3 seconds yields reliable SWI in the majority of patients. Based on other studies with a similar approach, if this interval is as long as 10 seconds (Peltola et al., 2014), it will probably lead to overestimation and an enhanced ceiling effect.

Besides the SWI, the same spike-detection algorithms can be used to calculate the number of spikes per unit of time. Even if in a certain range a linear relation exists between the two measures (Larsson et al., 2009), there is a substantial and conceptual difference between computing the "time occupied by epileptiform activities" (or "spike and wave index" [SWI]) *vs* the "number of spikes/unit of time" (or "Spike Frequency" [SF]). The SF has the advantage of avoiding the ceiling effect intrinsic to SWI calculation, particularly with paroxysmal discharges >60/min (Larsson et al., 2009; Sánchez-Fernández et al., 2012). The use of SF might only preclude comparison with the "classical" percentage thresholds used in the past (Cantalupo et al., 2013), and studies aiming to compare SF and SWI - in terms of their ability to correlate with the clinical condition - are lacking. In other words, it is unclear whether the linear SF measures or the SWI better reflects the clinical features of ESES.

Overall, the methods employing the automatic counting of individual spikes may lead to some important features being overlooked, such as fundamental intermittent focal pseudo-slowing, corresponding to a sequence of prominent slow waves following low-amplitude spikes (Massa et al., 2001).

SWI variability

SWI varies within and between patients. Within patients there are dynamic changes during the night (see below), but there are also variations from night to night (see also Gardella et al., p. 25-36). These variations are not well described and hence, not well understood. Reported between-patient variability ranges from 0 to 100%. *Figure 1* provides reported SWI values from 1913 recordings analyzed with a semi-automated method (Larsson et al., 2009). Cognitive impairment could be seen with SWI as low as 40. Probably, these low values are sufficient to produce negative influence in the brain. Anyway, in some cases, an underestimation of the SWI due to day-to-day variations cannot be excluded.

SWI also varies according to age of the subjects (*figure 2*). There is a tendency for a bell-shaped distribution with the highest values and the highest number of patients of around 10-11 years of age tapering off towards 18. This tapering is generally acknowledged to be due to puberty.

Caution should be taken interpreting this plot. At the left side, there is a time lag from symptoms until a full night EEG is recorded. There was no routine follow-up, and hence there are a set of reasons for recording in the middle of the age span. Also, the few recordings at the right side are probably influenced by the lack of new indications for a repeated recording.

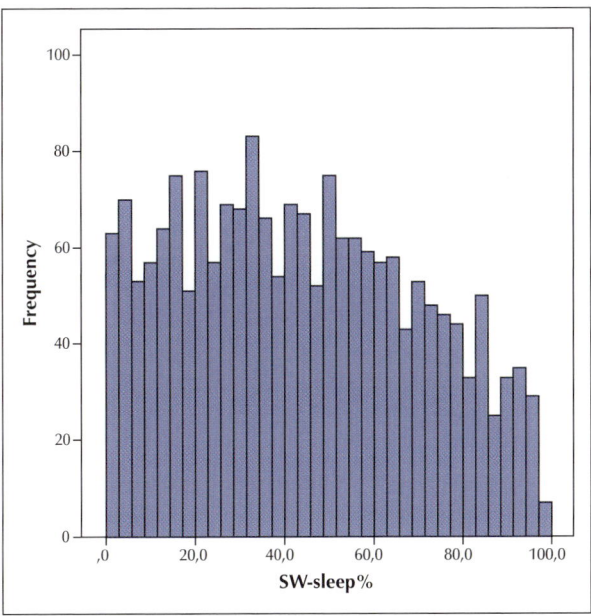

Figure 1/ Frequency distribution of SWI - computed according to Larsson et al., 2009 with max ISI=3 - based on 1913 consecutive recordings. The x-axis corresponds to SWI during sleep and the y-axis to the number of recordings within a given SWI interval. (Data from PGL).

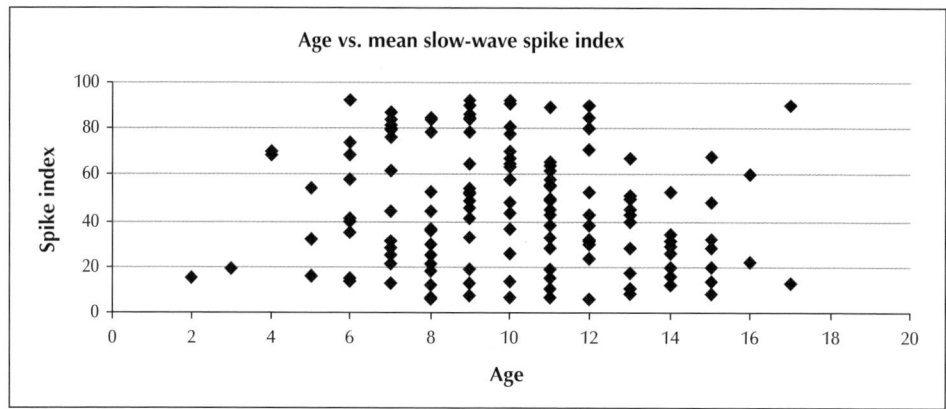

Figure 2/ Relation between age and spike index (computed according to Larsson et al. [2009] with max ISI=3) based on 132 full night recordings. (Data from PGL).

Time course

When referring to SWI, usually a single value is given, usually the mean. This can be sufficient when a uniform distribution of discharges across the entire recording is present. This is in agreement with the term "continuous spike-and-wave during slow sleep" (CSWS), implying that the pattern of diffuse spike-and-waves should be continuously present. However, this is true only in a subset of children, while a more fragmented or skewed pattern is the most common (*figures 3, 4*). In these latter cases, a single mean SWI value for each recording does not illustrate accurately the differences in temporal distribution of EEG abnormalities throughout the recording. This is particularly important in evaluating studies in which SWI is computed only based on a relatively brief EEG recording. In fact, even if

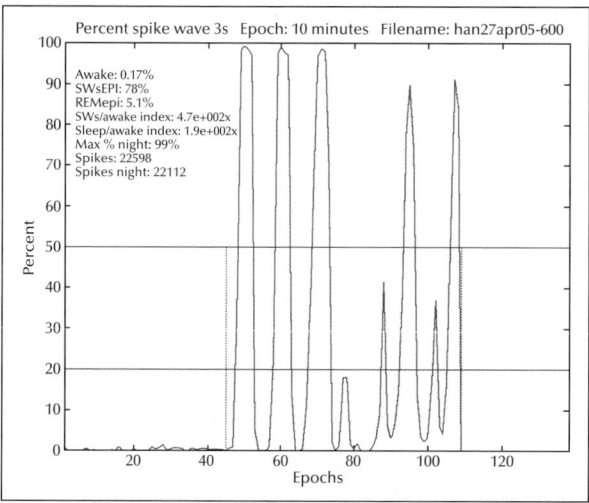

Figure 3/ SI (computed accordingly to Larsson et al. [2009] with max ISI=3) plotted in 10-minute epochs over 21 hours. The night sleep starts at about epoch 45. The dips in the plot reflect REM-sleep periods. SWI was reported as 78% for this patient. (Data from PGL).

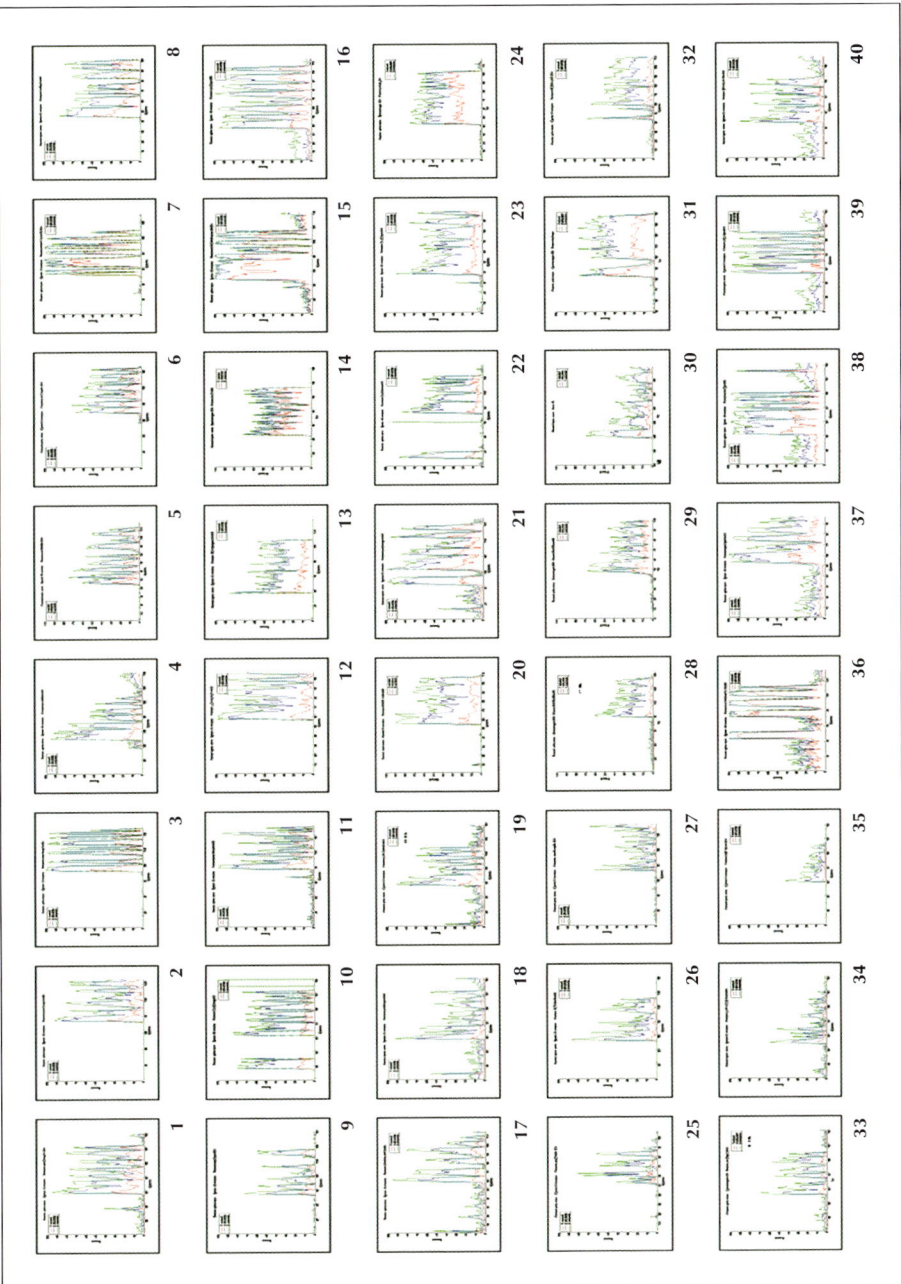

Figure 4/ SWI from 40 full night recording. The x-axis gives time in epochs (number for each 10th 10 minutes epoch). Y-axis gives SWI computed accordingly to Larsson et al. (2009). In the plot red, blue and green represents max ISI of 1, 3 and 5 seconds respectively. (Data from PGL).

it is clear that the "original" SWI is computed considering the entire nocturnal sleep EEG, the principal difference in subsequent studies reflects the proportion of the EEG recording analyzed. *Figure 4* provides an overview of 40 consecutive, full night recordings showing a wide range of patterns. In almost all recordings, a rhythm with a cycle time (close to 90 minutes) is seen, corresponding to sleep cycles.

Before the introduction of computer-aided techniques, the quantitative analysis of the entire overnight EEG was considered highly time-consuming and the majority of authors calculated the SWI based on a shorter EEG recording or a subsampling of the overnight EEG (see Scheltens-de Boer, 2009 for details). However, using a computer-aided semi-automated method like the one applied by Larsson *et al.* (2009) usually requires less than 30 minutes, mostly computer time, for the analysis of a full night recording.

During the era of analog EEG recording, the sleep EEG of a patient with ESES can be recognized just by looking at the very beginning of the EEG (*figure 5*). Although seemingly implausible or an over-simplification, this judgment is a statistical estimation based on scientific grounds: (1) the initial part represents a subsampling of the entire recording (one sample of about 10-20 ms for each 40-s folded page); (2) only high-amplitude spikes

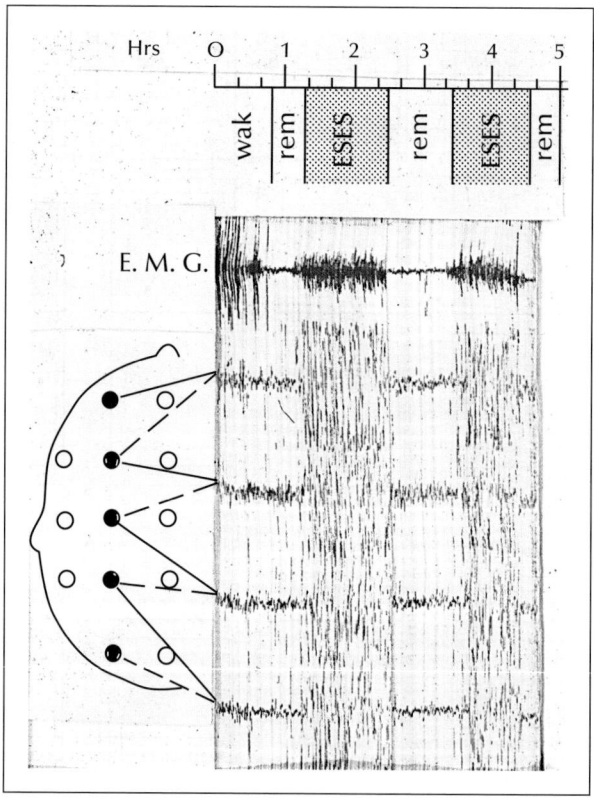

Figure 5/ In this archival image, the very beginning of a paper EEG tome is mounted beside an EEG montage scheme (left) and an ad-hoc time scale (upper) and different sleep stages are identified based on the corresponding pattern visible on the paper trace. During NREM sleep, the trace reflects the occurrence of almost continuous high-amplitude spike-and-waves of ESES. (Courtesy of prof. C.A. Tassinari - personal iconography).

or steep transients can be observed in such a limited time fraction; (3) the chance to view a high number of sequential high-amplitude spikes increases as the SI approximates to 100%, particularly when the time distribution is homogeneous. This was the case for the "classical" cases, however since the Venice Colloquium it was evident that these cases represented "the tip of the iceberg", in which the bulk is constituted by patients with similar clinical features but less EEG abnormalities (Beaumanoir, 1995). Particularly in those cases, a preferential occurrence of discharges in certain sleep stages can be observed. Nobili and coworkers (2001) demonstrated a higher number of discharges in the early stage of NREM sleep, but it should be noted that a prevalence in slow sleep can also be found (Cortinovis *et al.*, 1995), revealing that different distributions are possible (*figure 6*).

Looking at the variability of SWI across the night and in different sleep stages (*figure 6*), it is clear that the choice of the subsample will affect the results in a way that varies from one patient to another. In particular, analyzing only the onset of sleep or a nap EEG will give a reliable result in patients with a homogeneous distribution, but will probably overestimate the SWI in patients with a high number of abnormalities in the first cycle and few discharges in the latter cycles. The same is true regarding the sleep stages. Sampling the first 30 minutes of NREM sleep of the first and last sleep cycles (Aeby *et al.*, 2005) will mitigate the error due to the difference between sleep cycles but will not avoid the bias introduced by overestimating patients with high SWI in stages I-II (*figure 6B*) versus patients with the highest SWI in stage III-IV (*figure 6A*). This would also give erroneous results based on analysis of only one sleep-wake cycle (Saltik *et al.*, 2005), a 15-min slow wave sleep (Lewine *et al.*, 1999) or the first 5 minutes of NREM stage 2 during the first sleep cycle (Sánchez-Fernández *et al.*, 2012) or 100 seconds of sleep (Weber *et al.*, 2017). In fact, in patients with a large number of EDs (*i.e.* "classic" SWI >85%), there is good concordance between the traditional full-night method and "shortcut" methods used to analyse a small fraction of the night (Azcona *et al.*, 2017), however, we do not know the reliability of those "shortcut" methods in patients with an intermediate amount or inhomogeneous distribution of EDs. Similarly, although a correlation has been demonstrated between nap and overnight SWI (Larsson *et al.*, 2010), data from Dianalund Epilepsy Centre suggested that the two values can be discordant based on a non-negligible number of subjects (Gardella *et al.*, 2016). To overcome the drawback of a unique SWI value, Scheltens-de Boer (2009) proposed to express the SWI as mean, range and most encountered value. Other possible adjunctive measures are the standard deviation of SWI, the percentage of time spent over a certain threshold, the SWI for each sleep stage, and - probably the most informative - Area Under the Curve (AUC) for both SWI and SF.

Quality

Topography

It is now recognized that spike-and-waves characterizing ESES are actually focal or multifocal discharges with a more or less prominent phenomenon of propagations and projection (ranging from focal ESES to the classic one - see Gardella *et al.*, p. 25-36). A time course of amplitude mapping has been used to demonstrate that the generalized aspect of spike-and-waves is the result of the extreme propagation of focal abnormalities (Farnarier *et al.*, 1995), through the mechanism of secondary bilateral synchrony (Kobayashi *et al.*, 1994). Propagation of interictal EDs can be an indirect measure of the extent of

Figure 6/ Overnight variation of the level of EDs in three patients with ESES. Different patterns can be observed: (A) the "slow-sleep pattern", with few discharges during wakefulness and REM sleep and increasing EDs from sleep stage I-II to sleep stage III-IV; (B) the "light-sleep pattern" with maximal EDs during sleep stage II, paralleling the sigma power as described by Nobili *et al.* (2001); (C) the "continuous pattern" with almost no difference between REM and NREM sleep. In each panel, the upper line represents a hypnogram based on visual scoring (accordingly to Rechtschaffen and Kales, 1968). In the lower part of each panel, the graph is generated by means of homemade MATLAB scripts (The Mathworks, Natick, MA) using EEG spike recognition trough BrainVision Analyzer 2.0 software (Brain Products, Munich, Germany). Blue lines represent the Spike frequency (number of spike/minute) and red lines the SI calculated using Larsson's method (Larsson *et al.*, 2009) - using max ISI=3; one value/min. (Data from GC and PA).

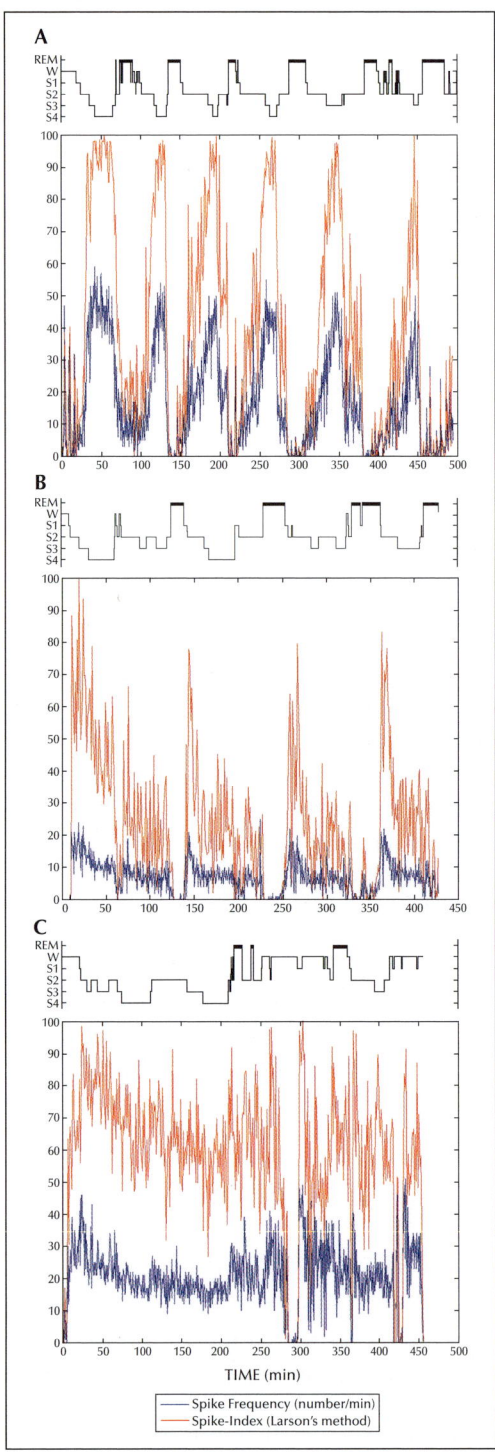

the "epileptic network". However, up to now only few studies extracted some quantitative objective and reproducible measures for this feature. One of the most interesting approaches used Electric Source Imaging with a distributed model to calculate the amplitude of primary source and the number of propagation regions (Larsson et al., 2010). Another fascinating methodology has been proposed recently by Peltola and coworkers (2014) to extract the "spike-strength" (SS), an amplitude-derived value expressing both the spatial extent and the density of synchronously acting neuronal networks. The latter measure has the great advantage of being possibly plotted over time, allowing a combined use with the time-course of SWI and/or SF. A limitation of SS with respect to Larsson's propagation measure is the reduced information about propagation at distant sites. A promising method can be the use of Independent Component Analysis to better extract the primary and propagated sources. In fact, by analyzing the temporal evolution of the averaged EDs projected onto the Independent Component space (for details see Abreu et al., 2015), we can observe the different components of the spike-and-wave complex as virtually separated EDs with millisecond delays (figure 7A). It would then be possible to compute SWI, SF, and SS for each component, providing more detailed topographic information of the most involved region in ESES.

High Frequency Oscillations

High frequency oscillations (HFOs) ranging from 80 to 500 Hz have been identified as possible biomarkers for epileptogenic tissue based on intracerebral recordings, but recently HFOs were described also on scalp EEG of patients with symptomatic and idiopathic ESES, including LKS (Kobayashi et al., 2010; Gong et al., 2018). The possibility to record HFOs from scalp indicates the presence of hypersynchronous pathological high-frequency activity that involves a relatively large cortical area (Kobayashi et al., 2010). These HFOs can be observed, with the appropriate filtering, in strict association with spikes, however, not all the spikes are associated with HFOs, even in the same patient and in the same recording (figure 7B, C). Based on clinical data, HFOs associated with spikes have been proposed as a potential negative prognostic marker in Idiopathic Focal Epilepsies of Childhood, indicating a possible evolution to ESES/CSWS (Kobayashi et al., 2011). Further studies confirmed that HFOs in patients with ESES might reflect disease activity and treatment response (Qian et al., 2016; Gong et al., 2018). Thus, in our opinion, the presence (and abundance) of spike-related HFOs could be another quantitative variable to be integrated into the evaluation of ESES.

Sleep

Sleep structure

Apart from epileptiform activities, the overnight EEG recordings allow the extraction of a number of sleep-related features, potentially useful for the evaluation of patients affected by ESES. Since the first descriptions of the syndrome, attention was payed to the presence or absence of sleep graphoelements (namely sleep spindles) and a recognizable sleep macrostructure, with alternating NREM/REM stages and succeeding sleep cycles (Patry et al., 1971; Beaumanoir, 1995).

Sleep researchers have developed different, reliable quantitative measures based on visual inspection or computer-aided analysis of EEG signal (Ferri et al., 2005; Iber et al., 2007;

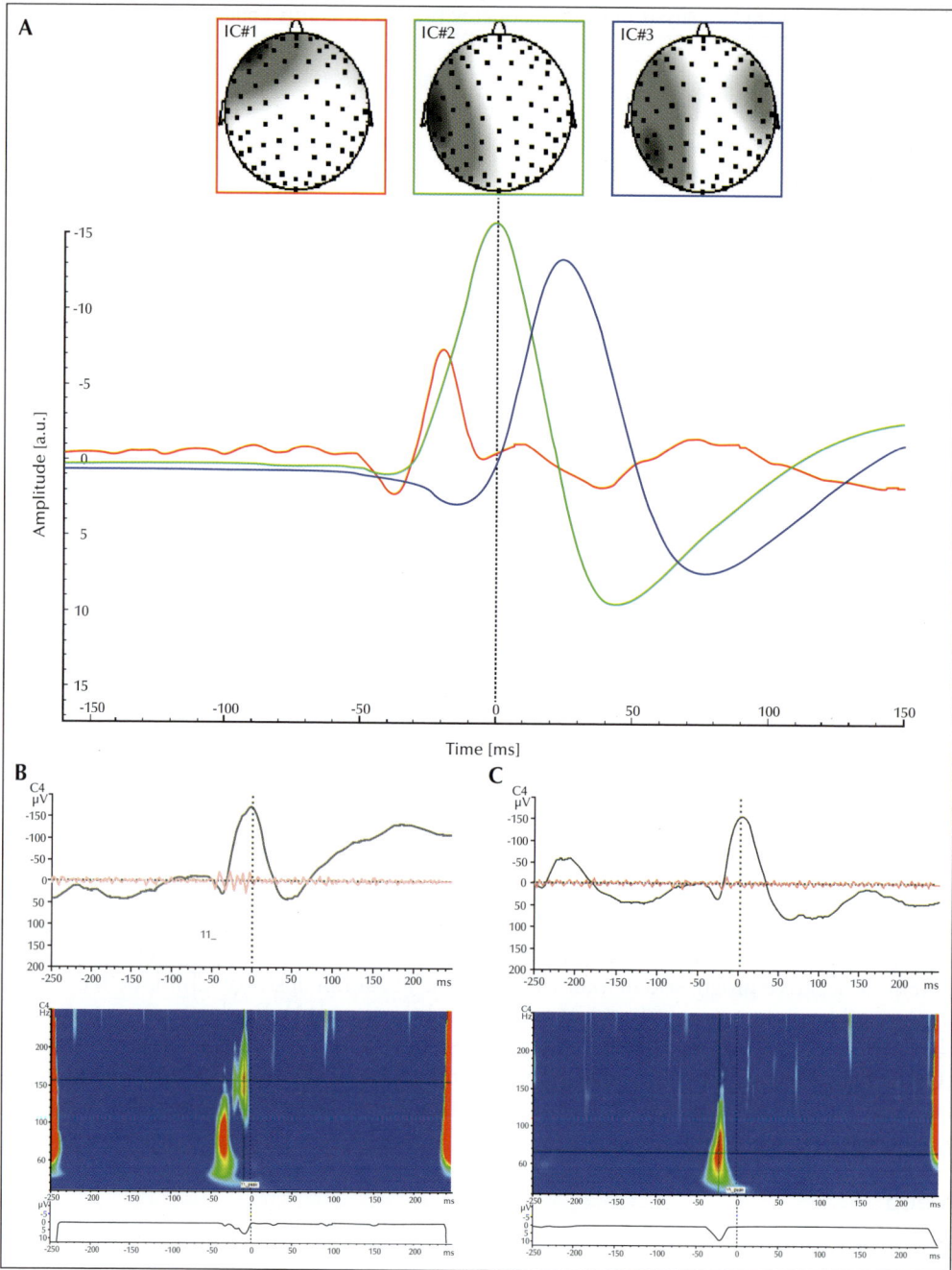

Figure 7/ (A) Example of Independent Component (IC) Analysis applied to decompose raw 128-channels EEG, containing bilateral spikes, apparently synchronous on right and left centro-temporal regions. Amplitude time course of the average spike projected onto the IC space allows the recognition of an early component (IC#1- red) with left frontal field, followed by the left centro-parietal component (IC#2- green; peaking 30 ms after IC#1) and the bilateral component (IC#3- blue; delayed by 30 ms from previous IC). Lower panels illustrate individual spikes from one subject - same topography and shape- with (B) or without (C) associated HFOs. In both panels a 500-ms time window centered on spike peak is represented. The upper part shows the unfiltered monopolar EEG (C4 channel) in black and the same EEG trace high-pass filtered above 100 Hz superimposed in red. The lower part represents the time-frequency wavelet analysis of the same unfiltered EEG trace, showing that in B the HFOs associated with the spike are visible as power increase at around 150 Hz. All transformations in this figure were performed using BrainVision Analyzer 2.0 software (Brain Products, Munich, Germany). (Data from GC and PA).

Achermann, 2009). These analyses may indicate the quality of sleep macrostructure and provide markers of fragmentation/instability in sleep microstructure. However, these quantitative analyses have been rarely applied to ESES and related conditions (Nobili et al., 2001; Bruni et al., 2010; Gibbs et al., p. 61-7).

Slow waves downscaling

One particular sleep-related EEG phenomenon deserves particular attention in the context of ESES (Tassinari et al., 2009). In fact, according to the synaptic homeostasis hypothesis (see also Rubboli et al., p. 69-76), the beneficial effects of sleep on brain function and performance is due to the progressive renormalization (downscaling) of synaptic strength occurring during sleep. A higher synaptic strength at sleep onset is reflected by a higher synchronization of large cortical areas that in turn are responsible for the generation of EEG Slow Wave Activity (SWA). An overnight decrease of the slope of individual Slow Wave from the first to the last hour of sleep, which parallels the decline in SWA in the course of sleep, is an indirect testimonial of the occurrence of the physiologic sleep-related synaptic downscaling (Vyazovskiy et al., 2009). Using this indirect quantitative measure, an alteration of the physiologic overnight decrease of the Slow Wave slope has been demonstrated in ESES (Bölsterli et al., 2011). This lack of SWA downscaling was evident only on the affected hemisphere in focal cases, and interestingly the degree of the impairment of the overnight slope decrease correlated with spike frequency (Bölsterli et al., 2014). Furthermore, recent evidence demonstrates that these alterations of overnight dynamic SWA during active ESES are reversible when ESES resolves (Bölsterli et al., 2017).

■ Conclusions

In conclusion, the diagnosis of Encephalopathy cannot be done based on EEG without clinical information and does not rely only on EEG (i.e. ESES is not solely an EEG pattern; see Cantalupo et al., 2013). A semiquantitative visual inspection, yielding an approximated amount of epileptiform abnormalities in overnight sleep EEG can be sufficient for diagnosis when a full-blown clinical picture is present (appearance or worsening of neurological, cognitive and/or behavioral disturbances). However, the challenge for clinicians is to recognize also very selective or subtle deficit possibly due to impairment of local SWA homeostasis induced by Status Epilepticus during Sleep (Tassinari et al., 2015). Up to now, there has been a lack of accurate and adequately powered studies on correlation between amount of epileptiform activity and neurocognitive regression. Moreover, the amount of EDs is only one of the potential and somewhat independent features that can be quantified in EEG recordings of ESES (see also Gardella et al., p. 25-36). Probably this is why currently there is no clear-cut lower boundary beyond which an EEG pattern is suggestive of evolution into ESES before the clinical diagnosis.

Possibly, an improved combination of clinical data and computer-aided EEG analysis will offer us the opportunity to recognize "dangerous" EEG features early in the course of the syndrome, thus to foresee (and possibly prevent) the evolution into ESES in patients at risk, but without an overt encephalopathy (Cantalupo et al., 2011; Tassinari et al., 2019). Thus, it is desirable that in future studies different EEG measures would be calculated in the same population (including ED amount, quality, and sleep-related features - such as macro-/micro-structure and SWA downscaling) in order to find out which (alone or in combination) is the best EEG correlate of clinical evolution.

■ Acknowledgements

This research was supported by the European Union Seventh Framework Programme FP7 under the project DESIRE (grant agreement 602531) to G.C.

Update on the genetics of the epilepsy-aphasia spectrum and role of *GRIN2A* mutations

Gaetan Lesca, Rikke S. Møller, Gabrielle Rudolf,
Edouard Hirsch, Helle Hjalgrim, Pierre Szepetowski

The so-called "idiopathic" childhood focal epilepsies (IFE) correspond to a broad spectrum of childhood epilepsy syndromes with specific age-dependent onset and typical EEG features such as multifocal spikes or spike-waves of various topographies. Childhood epilepsy with centro-temporal spikes (ECTS), also known as Rolandic epilepsy (RE), is the most frequent IFE. The relationships between RE and various comorbid manifestations and conditions, such as migraine, cognitive and behavioral issues, or reading impairment, have increasingly been recognized. Furthermore, the association with transient or permanent speech and/or language impairment has long been reported; hence the identification of the genetic syndrome of RE with verbal dyspraxia (Scheffer *et al.*, 1995). Epileptic Encephalopathy related to Status Epilepticus during slow Sleep (ESES) and Landau-Kleffner syndrome (LKS) -also known as 'acquired' epileptic aphasia - are two closely related epileptic encephalopathies (EEs) that represent more severe and less frequent forms of the IFE continuum. Indeed, all those syndromes are now considered different clinical expressions of the same pathological spectrum (Rudolf *et al.*, 2009). They all share the association of usually infrequent seizures with paroxysmal EEG discharges activated during drowsiness and sleep, sometimes fulfilling, in a subset of the patients, the criteria of status epilepticus during slow-wave sleep (SES), with more or less severe acquired neuropsychological and behavioral deficits.

■ General considerations about the genetic architecture of childhood focal epilepsies

A more modern view, that takes into account the recent advances in the genetic origin of various types of epilepsies, has recently challenged the classical distinction between idiopathic and symptomatic epilepsies (Berg *et al.*, 2010). Indeed, based on some of the many possible examples, it has somehow unexpectedly demonstrated that various types of EEs, such as the Dravet syndrome or the Ohtahara syndrome, can have simple, monogenic causes (Depienne *et al.*, 2012; Allen *et al.*, 2013). Conversely, epilepsies of genetic origin (formerly considered as 'idiopathic') can be associated with comorbid neurological conditions (*e.g.* migraine, behavioral or cognitive issues) or with structural lesions (*e.g.* cortical dysplasia). In the IFE, the possible existence of behavioral and cognitive issues, for instance, inherently challenged the use of the 'benign' term. It had long been assumed that in contrast to generalized epilepsies, most focal epilepsies are caused by lesions, infections, tumors, etc. and are hardly under genetic influence. Twin studies and familial concurrences then indicated that focal epilepsies could also be sustained by genetic factors (Ryan, 1995). As an example, the mapping and the subsequent identification of the first 'monogenic epilepsy' gene (*CHRNA4*) encoding a nicotinic acetylcholine receptor subunit was obtained for autosomal dominant nocturnal frontal lobe epilepsy (ADNFLE) (Steinlein *et al.*, 1995). Since then, several genes responsible for rare types of monogenic focal epilepsies have been identified (Berkovic *et al.*, 2006).

Familial aggregation has long been recognized in RE (Neubauer *et al.*, 1998). Relatives of RE patients display higher risk of epilepsy (notably RE, LKS or ESES) than control individuals (De Tiege *et al.*, 2006; Vears *et al.*, 2012; Dimassi *et al.*, 2014). Most RE, however, do not show a simple inheritance. In contrast to RE, the genetic influence in LKS and ESES has long remained controversial (Landau and Kleffner, 1957; Rudolf *et al.*, 2009) and a role for autoimmunity has even been hypothesized (Connolly *et al.*, 1999; Nieuwenhuis *et al.*, 2006). Recent advances in molecular cytogenetics and in next-generation DNA sequencing have dramatically helped in solving this issue. Consistent with the existence of genomic defects (copy number variations) that may have possible pathophysiological influence in numerous human disorders including the epilepsies (Helbig *et al.*, 2009; Mefford *et al.*, 2010), the screening of a series of 61 patients with LKS or ESES led to an overall picture with highly heterogeneous genomic architecture (Lesca *et al.*, 2012). A large number of potentially pathogenic alterations corresponded to genomic regions or genes (*e.g.* encoding cell adhesion proteins) that were either associated with the spectrum of autism disorders, or involved in speech or language impairment - which was of interest given the well-known association of LKS and ESES with autism-like manifestations (*e.g.* regression, disturbance of social interactions, perseveration) and with language disorders.

■ The role of *GRIN2A* mutations in RE/ESES/LKS

The study by Lesca and colleagues led to detection of several *de novo* genomic alterations including deletions of the NMDA glutamate receptor (NMDAR) subunit gene *GRIN2A* (Lesca *et al.*, 2012). Besides the obvious crucial function of NMDARs in the brain (Burnashev & Szepetowski, 2015), a few *GRIN2A* defects had previously been reported in patients with severe neurodevelopmental disorders (Reutlinger *et al.*, 2010; Endele *et al.*, 2010). Since then, the crucial and direct causal role of *de novo* or inherited *GRIN2A* mutations (microdeletions, splice-site, nonsense and missense mutations) in LKS, in ESES, and in RE with verbal dyspraxia has been demonstrated in three parallel studies (Carvill *et al.*, 2013; Lemke *et al.*, 2013; Lesca *et al.*, 2013). The mutations were found in all the different domains of the corresponding GluN2A (formerly known as NR2A) subunit, making it difficult to draw any clear genotype-phenotype correlation (Burnashev and Szepetowski, 2015; von Stülpnagel *et al.*, 2017). However, *de novo* mutations of *GRIN2A* might cluster in and around the ligand-binding sites and the transmembrane domains (Strehlow *et al.*, 2015).

The existence of a simple, unifying pathophysiological mechanism remains elusive: whereas the existence of microdeletions and nonsense mutations indicated loss-of-function (LOF) effects, some missense mutations seemed to lead to gain-of-function (GOF), at least *in vitro*, and some may even have multiple effects (Yuan *et al.*, 2014; Swanger *et al.*, 2016; Sibarov *et al.*, 2017). Interestingly, a recent study has indicated that some *GRIN2A*-associated EEs caused by gain-of-function mutations might be treatable by the NMDA receptor blocker, memantine (Pierson *et al.*, 2014). This study confers hope for more targeted therapeutic strategies in *GRIN2A*-related seizure disorders caused by GOF mutations. Nevertheless, an alteration in the Glun2B-to-GluN2A developmental switch, as suggested by altered kinetics of the mutant NMDARs (Carvill *et al.*, 2013; Lesca *et al.*, 2013), and a dysfunction of the thalamocortical network are likely. As a matter of fact, *Grin2a* knockout mice one month old, exhibit a series of transient brain microstructural alterations that involve the thalamus and the neocortex, and also display rare spontaneous epileptiform discharges in the third postnatal week (Salmi *et al.*, 2018). A case report suggested that the epileptic discharges could have a triggering role in the speech deterioration observed in children carrying a deleterious variant of *GRIN2A* (Sculier *et al.*, 2017).

Based on the initial studies, it has been estimated that up to 20% of patients with RE, LKS or ESES have a mutation in *GRIN2A*. A recent exome-wide study of the mutational burden in patients with typical and atypical RE showed that *GRIN2A* was the only gene with a significantly enriched burden associated with deleterious and LOF mutations (Bobbili *et al.*, 2018). However, interestingly, the statistical significance of this burden disappeared after excluding atypical RE patients, indicating that *GRIN2A* is more likely to cause phenotypes within the severe end of the disease spectrum (Bobbili *et al.*, 2018).

■ Other rare monogenic causes of ESES

Besides *GRIN2A*, other rare monogenic causes, particularly for ESES, have been reported (*table 1*). ESES has been reported in patients with LOF mutations in *KCNA2* encoding the potassium channel subunit $K_v1.2$. The patients usually present with febrile and multiple afebrile, often focal seizure types, multifocal epileptiform discharges strongly activated by sleep, mild to moderate intellectual disability, delayed speech development, and sometimes ataxia (Syrbe *et al.*, 2015; Masnada *et al.*, 2017). Interestingly, mutations in another potassium channel gene, *KCNB1*, have also been detected in patients with developmental and epileptic encephalopathies and an ESES-like pattern on the EEG (*figure 1*) (de Kovel *et al.*, 2017; Marini *et al.*, 2017).

Furthermore, several genetic and genomic defects of the *CNKSR2* gene, encoding an adaptor protein of the postsynaptic density, have been identified in patients with clinical features reminiscent of the epilepsy-aphasia spectrum (Lesca *et al.*, 2012; Vaags *et al.*, 2014; Damiano *et al.*, 2017). Last but not least, recent publications also suggest that ESES may be a frequent and underestimated feature in patients with Christianson syndrome, a severe neurodevelopmental disorder due to mutations in *SLC9A6*, encoding the endosomal solute carrier (Na K/H) exchanger 6 (NHE6) (Zanni *et al.*, 2014; Mathieu *et al.*, 2018).

■ Genetic susceptibility factors

16p11.2 microduplications encompassing *PRRT2* have not been identified in patients with RE or atypical RE (Dimassi *et al.*, 2014; Reinthaler *et al.*, 2014). *PRRT2* has been associated with a wide range of paroxysmal neurological disorders including infantile convulsions,

Table 1. Monogenic causes of RE/LKS/ESES.

	GRIN2A	KCNA2	KCNB1	SLC9A6	CNKSR2
Inheritance	Autosomal dominant	Autosomal dominant	Autosomal dominant	X-linked recessive	X-linked recessive
Functional effect	LOF, GOF	LOF	LOF	LOF	LOF
Seizure type	Focal motor seizures, GTCS, myoclonia, dyscognitive seizures	Febrile and multiple afebrile, often focal seizure types	Tonic, focal-clonic, myoclonia, spasms atypical absences, eyelid myoclonia	Absence, myoclonia, generalized seizures	Generalized or focal seizures
Clinical regression	+/-	No	+/-	Yes	Yes
Pharmacoresistant	No	No	Yes	Yes	No
Possible on sleep EEG	Centrotemporal spikes or ESES	Multifocal epileptiform discharges strongly activated by sleep/ESES	Multifocal or GS/PS strongly activated by sleep/ ESES	ESES	ESES
ID	Possible	Severe	Severe	Severe	Severe
Autistic features	Possible	Possible	Possible	Yes	NK

Abbreviations: LOF: loss of function, GOF: gain of function, ESES: Encephalopathy related to Status Epilepticus during slow Sleep, GS/PS: generalized spikes/polyspikes, NK: not known, GTCS: generalized tonic-clonic seizures

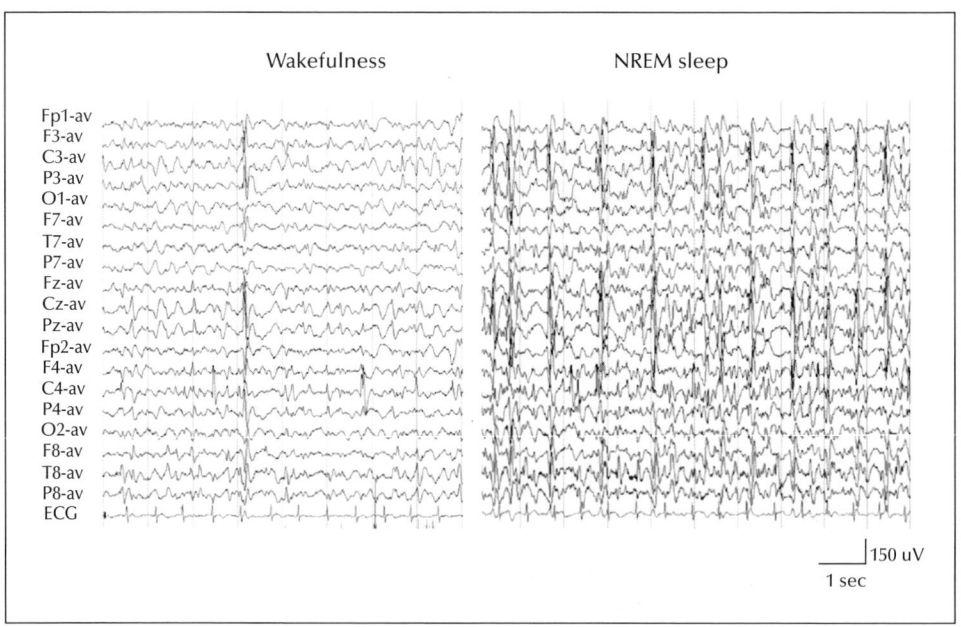

Figure 1/ Extreme activation of epileptic activity (spike-wave index during NREM sleep up to 98%) consistent with an ESES EEG pattern in a three-year-old boy with KCNB1 encephalopathy.

paroxysmal dyskinesia (mostly kinesigenic), or hemiplegic migraine (Cloarec et al., 2012; Lee et al., 2012), thus duplication of this gene may also confer risk for the development of RE.

Other potential genetic risk factors for RE have been suggested. For example, a dominant-negative rare variant previously identified in the *SRPX2* (Sushi-Repeat Protein, X-linked 2) protein (Roll et al., 2006) co-segregated with a p.Ala716Thr *GRIN2A* missense mutation in most affected members of a family with RE, verbal dyspraxia, and intellectual disability (Lesca et al., 2013). The *GRIN2A* mutation likely plays a key role in this family, although it had no obvious effect on a subset of NMDAR properties *in vitro* (Sibarov et al., 2017). On the other hand, *SRPX2* causes transcriptional down-regulation of *FOXP2* (Roll et al., 2010), which is associated with verbal dyspraxia (Lai et al., 2001). Furthermore, knockdown of *Srpx2 in utero* had dramatic consequences on neuronal migration in the developing rat cerebral cortex and led to postnatal epileptiform activity that was prevented by maternal administration of a tubulin deacetylase inhibitor (Salmi et al., 2013). Moreover, it was shown in mice that *Srpx2* also influences synaptogenesis and ultrasonic vocalization (Sia et al., 2013). Overall, rare *SRPX2* variants might correspond to genetic risk factors for various neurodevelopmental disorders; as a matter of fact, one splice-site *SRPX2* mutation was reported in a patient with autism (Lim et al., 2013), and the p.N327S rare variant was detected in a novel patient with LKS (Reinthaler et al., 2014).

Furthermore, *ELP4* has been proposed as a susceptibility gene for RE (Strug et al., 2009), however, this has never been confirmed. Mutations that might influence RE were also identified in the paralogous *RBFOX1* and *RBFOX3* neuronal splicing regulator genes (Lal et al., 2013), in the mammalian target of rapamycin regulator gene *DEPDC5* (Lal et al., 2014), and recently also in the *GABRG2* gene (Reinthaler et al., 2015).

■ Conclusion

In conclusion, several genes have been associated with LKS/ESES/RE, however, mutations in *GRIN2A* represent by far the most common genetic cause identified so far. As *GRIN2A* mutations unambiguously participate in the epilepsy-aphasia spectrum, whether and how genetic modifiers and environmental factors together with *GRIN2A* mutations contribute to the huge phenotypic variability, seen in the affected patients and families, emerges as an important question that surely deserves future investigation. Identification of other genetic and non-genetic factors and the ongoing studies with corresponding animal models, such as the *Grin2a* KO murine model, will help our understanding of the pathophysiology of this fascinating group of disorders situated at the crossroads between epileptic, cognitive, behavioral, and speech and language disorders.

■ Acknowledgements

This work was supported by ANR (Agence Nationale de la Recherche) grant 'EPILAND' (ANR-2010-BLAN-1405 01) with EuroBiomed label, by the National PHRC grant 2010 N° 03-08, by the European Union Seventh Framework Programme FP7/2007-2013 under the project DESIRE (grant agreement n°602531) and by INSERM (Institut National de la Santé et de la Recherche Médicale).

Pathophysiology of encephalopathy related to continuous spike and waves during sleep: the contribution of neuroimaging

Michael Siniatchkin, Patrick Van Bogaert

Epileptic encephalopathy with continuous spikes and waves during slow sleep (ECSWS) is an age-related disorder characterized by acquired variable neuropsychological impairment, epilepsy with heterogeneous seizure types, and the presence of the interictal electroencephalographic (EEG) findings of intense sub-continuous paroxysmal activity of spike-wave complexes that usually occupy more than 85% of non-REM sleep (Tassinari et al., 2005). ECSWS can be attributed to different etiologies (symptomatic cases with various structural brain lesions, and MRI-negative cases with probable genetic background, for example, in the form of Landau-Kleffner syndrome LKS or atypical benign partial epilepsy of childhood) and is associated in the majority of cases with manifold acquired psychomotor and cognitive deficits and even regressions (auditory agnosia, acquired aphasia, dysfunctions of the frontal lobe and short-term memory deficits, pseudo-bulbar palsy, global mental deterioration, impaired spatial orientation, apraxia and hemineglect, psychotic states and autistic features, attention deficit and hyperactivity and aggressiveness). Despite its significance, very little is known about pathophysiological mechanisms of ECSWS. Here, we summarize studies on functional neuroimaging which shed light on the pathophysiology of this defacing condition.

■ Source reconstruction

The first neuroimaging studies focused on the source reconstruction of epileptic spikes in patients with ECSWS and LKS based on EEG and MEG data. There is a general agreement that the perisylvian cortex is an important part of the network in patients with ECSWS (Morrell et al., 1995; Paetau et al., 1999; Sobel et al., 2000; Siniatchkin et al., 2010; Shirashi et al., 2014; De Tiege et al., 2013). In most cases with ECSWS, the perisylvian sources were found bilaterally, whereas in some patients with LKS, most sources were left-sided. The importance of the perisylvian cortex to trigger ECSWS is supported by clinical observations (frequent occurrence of ECSWS in patients with perisylvian polymicrogyria and association of structural abnormalities in the perisylvian region with LKS and ECSWS) and some treatment studies (encouraging results from multiple subpial transections in the perisylvian region in the treatment of ECSWS) (Morrell et al., 1995). It seems likely, however, that the perisylvian cortex is not always the generator of epileptic activity, even in patients with LKS (Paetau et al., 1999). In those cases where the generator is located in other cortical areas, the epileptic activity may propagate bilaterally to the perisylvian cortex (Morrell et al., 1995; Siniatchkin et al., 2010; De Tiege et al., 2013).

■ PET studies

The first PET studies were performed during sleep and wakefulness by Maquet et al. (1995) who investigated 6 patients with ECSWS of different etiology using [^{18}F]fluorodeoxyglucose (FDG). They showed unilateral, focal or regional cortical increases in glucose metabolism during both sleep and wakefulness. The most cortical areas associated with CSWS included perisylvian, superior temporal and inferior parietal areas. The metabolism in the cortical mantle was higher than in the subcortical regions. Interestingly, after successful treatment of ECSWS and recovery of symptoms, the described metabolic changes disappeared. The study of Maquet et al. provided important insight into the pathophysiology of ECSWS and enabled the following conclusions which were supported later by other studies:

- It seems likely that the associative cortex, especially the perisylvian and superior temporal regions, are involved in the generation and propagation of epileptic activity in CSWS. Although the study provides strong evidence for an individual focal cerebral dysfunction in CSWS, systemic abnormalities such as pathological activity in the thalamo-cortical network may play a significant role in this pathological condition.

- Similar metabolic changes in the brain may be found during sleep and in wakefulness. This fact may explain why patients with dramatic activation of epileptic activity during sleep develop cognitive deficits during the day, when the epileptic activity is less pronounced or may even disappear.

- The described pathological changes represent a functional fingerprint of ECSWS, independent of etiology.

These results were confirmed by the Brussels group in a number of publications. In these studies, data were analysed using a voxel-based statistical methodology that enabled group analyses and connectivity studies in addition to individual analyses. De Tiege et al. (2004) investigated 18 patients with ECSWS during wakefulness using FDG-PET and analyzed data at the individual level and at the group level using a group control of healthy young adults. At the individual level, they found areas of hypermetabolism in the cerebral cortex, clearly well associated with the focus of interictal epileptic activity. At the group level, hypermetabolic areas involved the postcentral gyrus and parietotemporal junction very close to the perisylvian region. In addition, areas of hypometabolism were found in most cases in the prefrontal and frontal cortex. Also at the group level, altered functional connectivity was found between hypermetabolic (parietal) and hypometabolic (frontal) brain regions and was interpreted as reflecting remote inhibition of frontal areas through epileptic activity as a possible explanation for cognitive deficits in affected individuals. These data were recently confirmed using a pediatric population as pseudo-controls, showing at the group level hypometabolism in regions that belong to the default network (prefrontal and posterior cingulate cortices, parahippocampal gyrus and precuneus) (Ligot et al., 2014). Later, De Tiege et al. (2008) investigated nine patients with ECSWS during the acute phase of the disease and recovery. Again, the authors described areas of focal hypermetabolism in the centro-parietal regions and right fusiform gyrus and widespread hypometabolism in the prefrontal and orbitofrontal cortices, temporal lobes, left parietal cortex, precuneus and cerebellum. Both hyper- and hypometabolism markedly regressed at recovery. These studies provided the evidence that the metabolic effects of CSWS activity and its associated neuropsychological impairments are not restricted to the epileptic foci but spread via the inhibition of remote neurons within connected brain areas. Finally, De Tiege et al. (2013) combined FDG-PET and source reconstruction in six patients with ECSWS. The areas of hypermetabolism were associated with the onset or propagation site of epileptiform discharges as revealed by the source analysis. Areas of hypometabolism were not related to epileptic activity.

Recently, Agarwal et al. (2016) studied glucose metabolism in 23 children with CSWS using FDG-PET with a specific focus on metabolic changes in the thalamus. Thalamic glucose metabolism was abnormal in 78,3% of patients. However, the abnormalities were very inhomogeneous. Some children were characterized by unilateral, some by bilateral, metabolic abnormalities, some of them demonstrated abnormal increases and some children showed decreases in metabolism. There was no clear association between thalamic metabolic abnormalities and the stage of evolution of ECSWS (prodromal, acute, or residual). Although determining the relevance of thalamic metabolic abnormalities in the pathogenesis of CSWS for any particular patient is challenging, the study emphasizes the role of thalamic pathology and significance of thalamo-cortical network in mechanisms of ECSWS (Agarwal et al., 2016).

In summary, PET studies have provided evidence for typical functional brain abnormalities in patients with ECSWS which (1) are characterized by the association with cortical focal hypermetabolism and hypometabolism in distinct connected cortical areas (the significance of thalamo-cortical network was underlined in several studies), (2) remain to be stable during wakefulness and sleep, and (3) are largely reversible at recovery of ECSWS, indicating that these abnormalities are attributed to epileptic activity. It is unclear whether these abnormalities are related to the increase of epileptic activity during sleep. One possible way to investigate this question is to study correlations between epileptiform discharges and neurometabolic / haemodynamic changes in the brain using simultaneous recordings of EEG and functional MRI (EEG-fMRI).

■ EEG-fMRI studies

The first EEG-fMRI study on CSWS was published by De Tiege et al. (2007). The authors investigated a nine-year-old girl suffering from partial seizures and who developed CSWS and neuropsychological deficits. Epileptiform activity was associated with focal activation in the right superior frontal, postcentral, and superior temporal cortex as well as deactivation in the lateral and medial frontoparietal cortices, posterior cingulate gyrus and cerebellum. In concordance with this study, Siniatchkin et al. (2010) investigated 12 children with ECSWS of different etiologies using simultaneous recordings of EEG and fMRI. The study revealed a typical network of brain activation in patients: the positive BOLD signal changes involved the bilateral perisylvian region (which was clear based on PET and MEG/EEG studies) and cingulate gyrus as well as bilateral frontal and parietal cortex and thalamus. Electrical source analysis demonstrated a similar involvement of the perisylvian brain regions, independent of etiology and area of spike generation. Moreover, the source reconstruction provided evidence that the typical pattern of brain activation is more likely to be related to a specific pattern of propagation of epileptic activity during ECSWS (*figure 1*). Negative BOLD signal changes were identified in the precuneus, lateral parietal cortex and medial frontal cortex. These structures are usually involved in a pattern of deactivation that occurs during the initiation of task-related activity and represent a default mode network (DMN) which is active in the resting brain with a high degree of functional connectivity (Raichle *et al.*, 2001). It has been suggested that the DMN constitutes a necessary favourable neurometabolic environment for cognitive functions, represents a physiological baseline for processes of attention and working memory, and supports dynamic integration of cognitive and emotional processing (Raichle and Mintun, 2006). Abnormal activity in the DMN and disturbed connectivity between the structures involved may influence task performance and contribute to pathogenesis of neuropsychiatric disorders such as attention-deficit hyperactivity, Alzheimer's disease, autism, schizophrenia, and depression (Broyd *et al.*, 2009). It has been suggested that disruption of the resting state activity by pathological processes (e.g. those that give rise to spikes) may be related to alterations in cognitive function and this may be a possible mechanism which may underlie cognitive deficits in epilepsy (Gotman *et al.*, 2005). Deactivation in the DMN has been described in patients with primary and secondary generalized paroxysms and absence seizures as well as in patients with temporal lobe epilepsy (for a review, see Moeller *et al.* [2013]). The authors hypothesized that one of the possible mechanisms to explain how epileptic activity in patients with ECSWS causes cognitive deficits is the mechanism of interruption of the activity and connectivity in the DFM. Note that areas of hypometabolism revealed by PET studies resemble those of deactivation in EEG-fMRI studies representing remote inhibition of the default mode network (Ligot *et al.*, 2014). This is an elegant hypothesis to explain cognitive deficits by inhibition/deactivation in the DMN. However, this hypothesis should be supported by neuropsychological and neuroimaging data, which has not yet been performed.

■ Functional and effective connectivity

There is another explanation for the interaction between the DMN and epileptic activity. Based on analysis of effective connectivity in patients with absence epilepsy, Vaudano *et al.* (2009) provided evidence that activity in the precuneus, as part of the DMN, gates spike-and-wave discharges in the thalamo-cortical network. It seems likely that haemodynamic changes in the precuneus, as an index of awareness and fluctuations of vigilance, trigger epileptic paroxysms (Vaudano *et al.*, 2009). The question whether the epileptic network causes changes in the DMN or vice versa was explored in the recent study of Japaridze *et al.* (2016). Sleep EEGs before and after treatment were investigated in fifteen patients with ECSWS (including three patients with Landau-Kleffner syndrome). In order to study functional and effective connectivity within the network generating the delta activity in background sleep EEG, the methods of dynamic imaging of coherent sources (DICS, a method of source analysis in frequency domain) and renormalized partial directed coherence (RPDC, a measure of causality between sources of activity) were applied. Independent of etiology and severity of epilepsy, the background EEG pattern in patients with ECSWS before treatment was associated with the complex network of coherent sources in the medial prefrontal cortex, somatosensory association cortex/ posterior cingulate cortex,

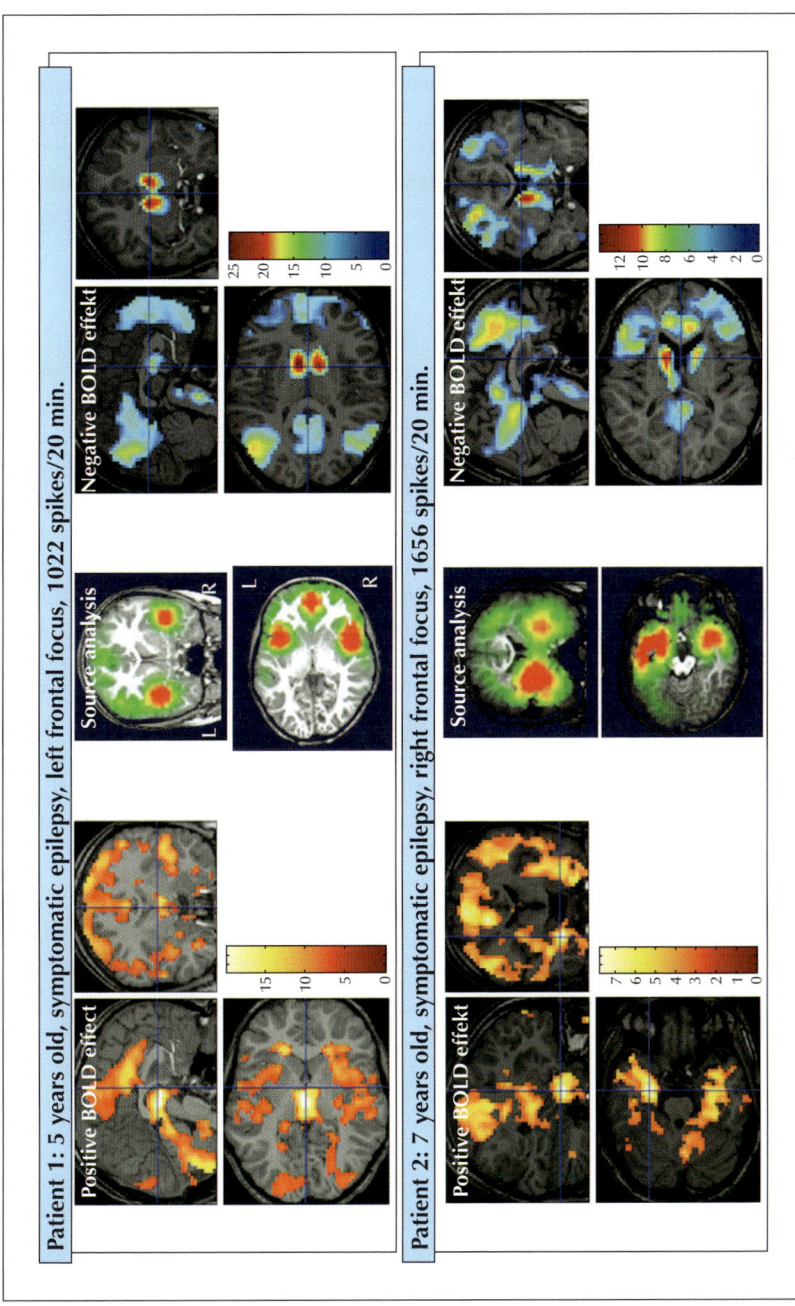

Figure 1/ Results of EEG-fMRI and of EEG source analysis in two patients with CSWS. (For methodological details see Siniatchkin *et al.* [2010].)

medial prefrontal cortex, middle temporal gyrus/ parahippocampal gyrus/ insular cortex, thalamus, and cerebellum (based on both individual as well as group level). The analysis of information flow within this network revealed the medial parietal cortex and precuneus as well as thalamus as central hubs, driving the information flow to other areas, especially to the temporal cortex where epileptic activity originates. The described CSWS-specific pattern of functional and effective connectivity was no longer observed in patients with normalized sleep EEG after a successful treatment. The study demonstrates the leading role of the precuneus and thalamus in the hierarchical organization of the network underlying the background EEG in CSWS and points towards the significance of fluctuations of vigilance in the generation of CSWS. This hierarchical network organization seems to be specific for CSWS as it resolves after successful treatment (Japaridze et al., 2016).

■ Conclusions

Functional neuroimaging represents a powerful methodology to investigate pathogenic mechanisms of epileptic encephalopathies including ECSWS. Recent studies demonstrated that in patients with ECSWS, different etiological factors correlate with the same pattern of network activation in areas including the perisylvian region, temporal, parietal and cingulate cortex. It seems likely that this CSWS-specific network represents a pattern of propagation of epileptic activity. Moreover, besides the network related to epileptiform discharges, there are changes in brain activity remote from the epileptic focus. These remote areas of reduction of brain activity include the precuneus, parietal and medial frontal cortex - brain areas of the default mode network. It could be that the epileptic activity interferes with the DMN and, in such a way, influences cognitive function. According to this hypothesis, the remote inhibition may possibly explain cognitive deficits in patients with CSWS. However, it could also be that the fluctuation of activity in the DMN facilitate generation of epileptiform discharges. This hypothesis would explain an increase of epileptic activity during sleep in patients with CSWS. The described abnormalities are functional in nature and disappear after recovery of symptoms following successful treatment. Whatever the explanation, confirmatory studies are needed in order to explore the interaction between epileptic and other functional networks in patients with ECSWS.

Interictal epileptiform discharges in sleep and the role of the thalamus in Encephalopathy related to Status Epilepticus during slow Sleep

Steve A. Gibbs, Lino Nobili, Péter Halász

Sleep consists of repetitive cycles where NREM and REM sleep alternate with a periodicity of about 90-100 minutes. Each state requires distinctive regulatory mechanisms and exerts a different modulatory effect on physiologic and epileptic activity (Amzica, 2002; Brown et al., 2012). In this article, we will review the effect of sleep on interictal epileptic discharges (IEDs) with a particular attention on the activation and modulation of IEDs in the syndrome of Encephalopathy related to Status Epilepticus during slow Sleep (ESES). Finally, we will discuss the role of the thalamus and the cortico-thalamic circuitry in this syndrome.

■ Activation of IEDs during sleep

Scalp EEG studies have shown that NREM sleep increases the number of IEDs and favours seizure occurrence both in focal and generalized epilepsies while REM sleep does not (Ferrillo et al., 2000; Herman et al., 2001; Campana et al., 2017). NREM sleep can also facilitate the spread of IEDs, both ipsilaterally and contralaterally from the primary focus in focal epilepsy (Malow et al., 1998; Sammaritano et al., 1991), especially during arousal fluctuations, namely phase A of the cyclic alternating pattern (CAP) (Halász et al., 2004; Parrino et al., 2006). Conversely, this phenomenon is not observed in REM sleep, where a reduced spatial and temporal summation of electrical signals is observed, thereby limiting the propagation and scalp EEG expression of the IEDs (Sammaritano et al., 1991; Frauscher et al., 2016; Campana et al., 2017).

The mechanisms by which NREM sleep activates IEDs have been extensively studied since the original publication by Gibbs and Gibbs on the usefulness of sleep to record IEDs (Gibbs and Gibbs, 1947). Experimental data have demonstrated that the same physiological thalamocortical and cortical oscillations operating during NREM sleep and leading to the appearance of the typical physiological graphoelements (e.g. spindles and K complexes) also favour the occurrence of IEDs. In particular, the presence, during NREM sleep, of a continuous alternation between neuronal depolarization (up-state or activated state) and hyperpolarization (down-state or silent state) at the cellular level creates a state of instability that enables the epileptogenic cortical substrate to produce IEDs (Steriade et al., 1993; Amzica, 2002). Intra-cerebral sleep EEG recordings in epileptic patients have confirmed these findings showing that IEDs are modulated by cortical sleep slow waves being significantly more frequent during the transition from up to down state (Frauscher et al., 2015). Moreover, the presence of infraslow oscillations, as observed by both quantified and visual EEG analysis, seem to further increase the occurrence and the spread of IEDs by creating an additional instability operating at a macroscopic level (Vanhatalo et al., 2004; Halász et al., 2013; Gibbs et al., 2015; Zubler et al., 2017). Accordingly, Ujma et al. showed that IEDs recorded with subdural electrodes were maximally associated with phase A1 of the CAP (Ujma et al., 2015). Finally, these observations have been confirmed by Stereo-EEG studies, showing that the lowest level of IED production is observed during the plateau of delta activity, corresponding to a stable and spatially homogeneous production of delta activity in different brain regions (Gibbs et al., 2016; Zubler et al., 2017).

■ Activation and modulation of IEDs during sleep in ESES

ESES provides perhaps the most spectacular example of EEG activation of IEDs during sleep. The peculiar characteristic of this epileptic syndrome is state dependency. In wakefulness, the EEG is usually abnormal, showing paroxysmal foci in the fronto-temporal or centro-temporal regions or isolated bursts of diffuse spike-wave activity. During NREM sleep, an EEG pattern of nearly continuous, pseudo-rhythmic bursts of diffuse IEDs arises. This pattern typically stops upon entering REM sleep where IEDs become fragmented, less continuous and more localized (Tassinari et al., 2019). The shape and field potentials of IEDs in ESES show similarities with the IEDs of other childhood focal epilepsy syndromes such as benign epilepsy with centro-temporal spikes (BECTS), Panayiotopoulos syndrome (PS), atypical BECTS and Landau-Kleffner syndrome (LKS). Although IEDs are often bilateral, in ESES, as in these other syndromes, a leading hemisphere usually drives the IEDs with different degree of secondary bilaterality during sleep (Halász et al., 2005). Because of clinical and EEG similarities between ESES and these syndromes, it is therefore argued that ESES is at the far end of this continuum of syndromes. Indeed, BECTS, PS, atypical BECTS, LKS and ESES share a similar perisylvian location of IEDs, an important increase in IEDs during sleep, a deterioration of language and executive functions of various intensities as well as common genetic mutations (De Negri, 1997; Doose et al., 2001; Hahn et al., 2001; Halász et al., 2005; Panayiotopoulos et al., 2008; Lemke et al., 2013; Lesca et al., 2013; Turner et al., 2015). Sleep-related IED activation in ESES is henceforth thought to represent an extreme exaggeration of what is seen in BECTS during sleep, both in space and synchronicity (De Negri, 1997; Halasz et al., 2014).

Earlier EEG studies based on visual sleep stage scoring in patients with BECTS had identified slow wave sleep has a potent activator of IEDs (Beaumanoir et al., 1974; Dalla Bernardina et al., 1982; Clemens and Majoros, 1987), with the descending slope of the cycles having the greatest activating properties (Clemens and Majoros, 1987). By using spectral EEG analysis methods to compare IED dynamics on EEG plotted with temporal series of SWA, the main indicator of sleep depth, or spindle frequency activity (SFA), it was shown that a higher correlation between IED distribution and SFA with respect to SWA exists in

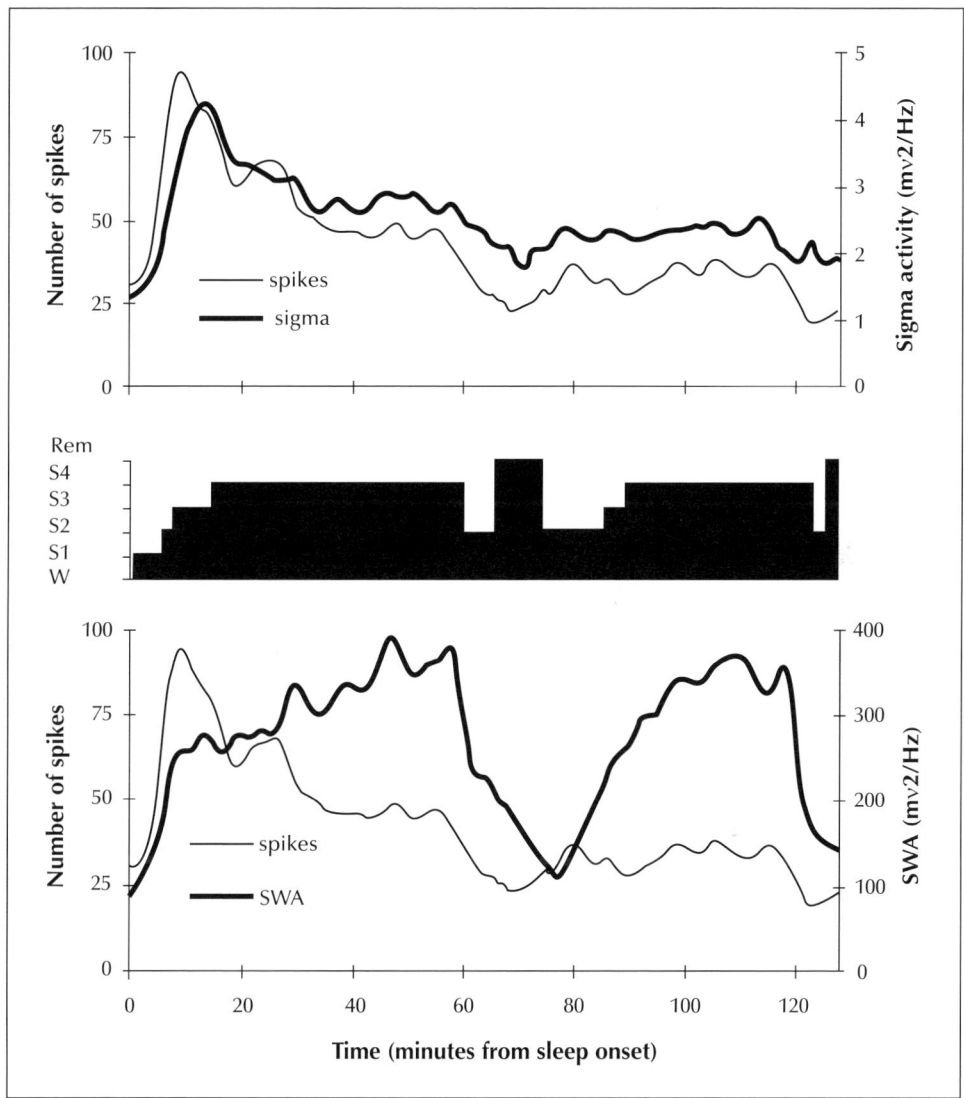

Figure 1/ Temporal series of spikes per minute plotted together with spindle frequency activity (sigma activity; upper graph) and slow-wave activity (SWA; lower graph) in a patient affected by Landau-Kleffner Syndrome. Hypnogram is shown in the center. Notice the better temporal relation between spikes per minute and spindle frequency activity with respect to SWA. Modified with permission from Nobili et al., 2000.

BECTS, PS, LKS and ESES (Nobili et al., 1999, 2000, 2001; Beelke et al., 2000) (*figure 1*). This finding differs from what is observed in adults with focal epilepsy, where IEDs are known to be strongly modulated by arousal fluctuations (CAP) (Terzano et al., 1991). Indeed, Terzano et al. have shown that IEDs in BECTS were not modulated by the CAP (Terzano et al., 1991). Moreover, when limiting the analysis to the part of the first NREM sleep cycle where SWA and SFA show a diverging behaviour (SWA increases and SFA decreases), Ferrillo et al. (2000) showed that correlation coefficients between SFA and

IEDs in childhood focal epilepsy syndromes were highly positive while correlations between SWA and IEDs were always negative, implying the existence of mutually exclusive sleep-related IEDs facilitating mechanisms.

In ESES, the tremendous amount of IEDs hinders the application of spectral EEG analysis. However, the cyclic organization of sleep in ESES is grossly preserved showing a standard ultradian rhythm with approximately 80% of total sleep time spent in NREM sleep versus 20% in REM sleep (*figure 2; upper panel*). This has permitted Nobili et al. to compare the physiological evolution of SWA and SFA EEG power in control subjects to the time series of IEDs in children with ESES (Nobili et al., 2001). Since SWA distribution is characterized by an exponential decay from the first to the last NREM sleep cycle during the night, one could hypothesize that a similar decay in IED production should occur throughout the night. However, as shown in *figure 2 (upper panel)*, the mean IED count did not change throughout the consecutive NREM cycles. Correlation analysis showed that the temporal distribution of IEDs was also positively correlated with SFA (*figure 2; lower panel*). This finding suggests that the IED activation throughout the night in ESES seems to be more sensitive to the sleep-promoting and -maintaining mechanisms than to the homeostatic process related to sleep depth.

Data on IED frequency extracted from the aforementioned studies are summarized in *table 1*. Values of IED frequency during NREM sleep show a constant increase from "benign" focal epilepsy syndromes to ESES. Of note, this progression also mirrors the clinical continuum of language and executive function deterioration observed in some of these children. Indeed, a peculiar aspect of these epileptic syndromes is their exclusive occurrence during a specific developmental period, from 2-14 years, an age when cortical synaptogenesis, abundant axonal sprouting and elemental functional network are being established (De Negri, 1997; Panayiotopoulos et al., 2008; Kurth et al., 2010). The abundance of IEDs during NREM sleep has lead to the hypothesis that excessive IEDs interfere with SWA production and/or modulation thus impeding the recuperating, downscaling and learning properties of slow wave sleep (see Rubboli et al., p. 69-76). It is also interesting to note, as evidenced in *table 1*, that an increase in IEDs is observed not only during NREM sleep but also during REM sleep, especially in LKS and ESES where the spike index remains very high during this state. In the future, further assessment of these phenomena might improve our understanding of the neuro-developmental deficits in ESES and more precisely the impact of IED frequency in different sleep states.

■ ESES: does the thalamus play a role?

The nature of IEDs in ESES during NREM sleep seems to be strongly linked to the cortico-thalamic circuitry. Patry et al. speculated that a "particularly active synchronizing system… could account for the extreme activation of the spike and wave discharges" (Patry et al., 1971). Although it is unlikely that the IEDs initiate in the thalamocortical circuit as once thought, this system is certainly implicated in its activation, apparently promoting and/or maintaining their occurrence, especially in the context of an immature hyperexcitable brain. Indeed, the observed correlation between IEDs and SFA in ESES seems to suggest that the same thalamocortical oscillations responsible for spindle occurrence create a neurophysiological substrate that favours the activation and spread of IEDs in an hyperexcitable immature cortex. Therefore, although the cortex is the minimum substrate

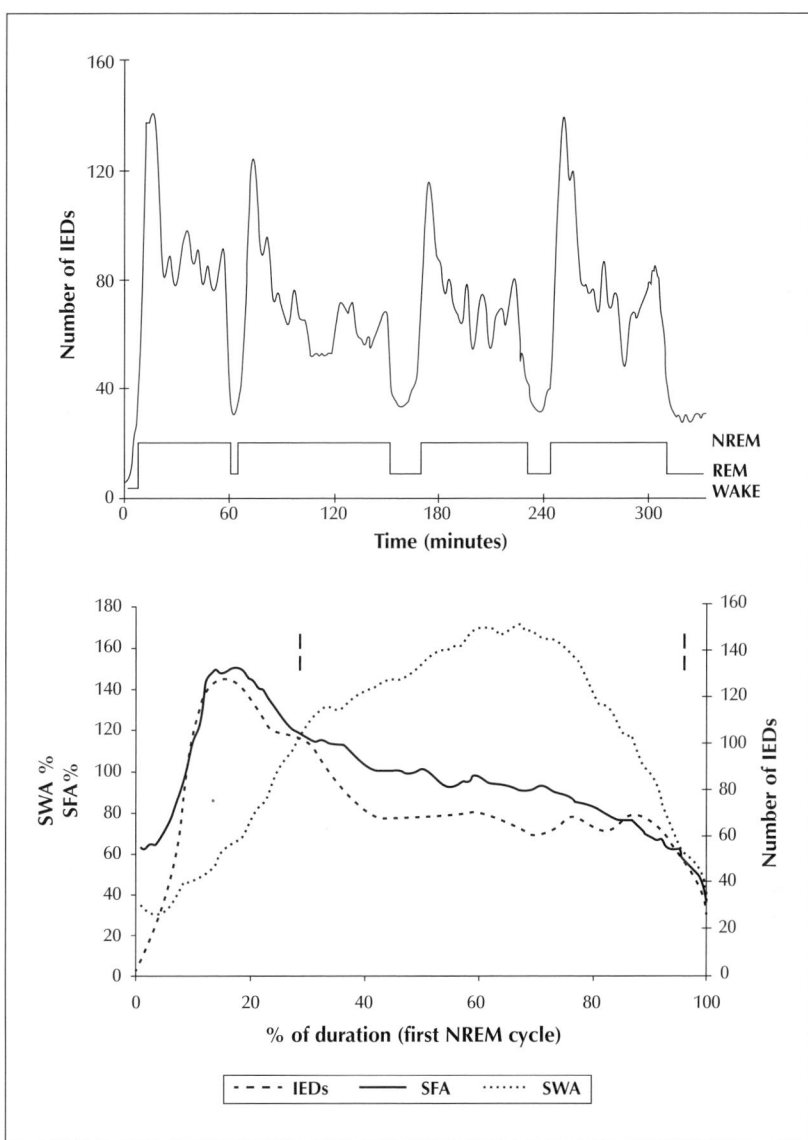

Figure 2/ Upper panel - temporal distribution of spikes during the whole night in a single representative subject with ESES. Notice the rather stable values of IEDs over the consecutive cycle. The hypnogram is shown under the IED profile. Lower panel - Model of normalized SWA and SFA time course in the first NREM sleep cycle in ESES. The distribution of IEDs per minute in a single subject shows a strong correlation with SFA and an inverse time course with respect to SWA, especially between the two dotted vertical lines where SFA and SWA have diverging behavior. ESES, Encephalopathy related to Status Epilepticus during slow Sleep; IEDs, interictal epileptiform discharges; SFA, spindle frequency activity; SWA, slow wave activity. Modified with permission from (Nobili et al., 2001).

Table 1. Spike index comparison during NREM and REM sleep in different syndromes of focal childhood epilepsy

	No. subjects	Age	NREM spike index	REM spike index
BECTS	9	7.4 (2.5)	23.5 (9.8)	6.3 (4.4)
PS	5	5.8 (2.1)	32.8 (12.3)	16.1 (8.6)
LKS	3	4.3 (0.5)	40.6 (5.6)	21.6 (3.8)
ESES	5	5.6 (1.1)	69.6 (10.1)	34.2 (4.7)

Spike index: number of spikes/minute; parenthesis: standard deviation; BECTS: benign epilepsy with centrotemporal spikes; PS: Panayiotopoulos syndrome; LKS: Landau-Kleffner; ESES: electrical status epilepticus during sleep. Data extracted from Beelke *et al.*, 2000; Nobili *et al.*, 2001, 2000, 1999.

necessary for the production of IEDs, connectivity of thalamic structures seems to have a role in their synchronization and spread (Steriade and Contreras, 1995). Once the oscillation has been set in motion, the cortex and thalamus is hypothesized to form a unified oscillatory network in which both structures drive each other (Meeren *et al.*, 2005). Using positron emission tomography with [18F]-fluorodeoxyglucose (FDG-PET) to study functional changes in cortical and thalamic metabolism, most studies found no significant or asymmetric metabolic changes in thalamic nuclei, therefore downplaying the role of the thalamus in ESES (Maquet *et al.*, 1995; De Tiège *et al.*, 2013, 2008). However, recent data suggest that reduced thalamic volume and hypo- or hypermetabolism can be observed in ESES, highlighting the complexity of studying this dynamic process (Agarwal *et al.*, 2015; Sánchez Fernández *et al.*, 2017).

The decrease or absence of metabolic changes in the thalamus does not, however, equate to thalamic silence. Using functional MRI (fMRI) analysis in a child with atypical BECTS and linguistic difficulties, Mirandola *et al.* highlighted the involvement of a wide cortico-subcortical network that involved the thalamus during sleep IEDs (Mirandola *et al.*, 2013). Such a thalamic involvement was absent during wake IEDs, in line with the role of spindle-generating mechanisms, favouring the activation and propagation of IEDs during sleep through secondary bilateral synchrony (Morrell *et al.*, 1995; Nobili *et al.*, 1999, 2001). A thalamic involvement during sleep-related IEDs has also been shown in some children with ESES (Siniatchkin *et al.*, 2010).

Another intriguing association between ESES and the thalamus concerns early thalamic lesions which have been suggested to play a role in generating ESES by damaging the thalamocortical circuit (Monteiro *et al.*, 2001; Leal *et al.*, 2018). Cohorts of children with early acquired thalamic injury have shown that approximately a third of these children go on to develop ESES (Veggiotti *et al.*, 1998; Monteiro *et al.*, 2001; Guzzetta *et al.*, 2005; Sánchez Fernández *et al.*, 2012). However, most reports linking thalamic injuries to sleep EEG activation and ESES concern children with extensive brain damage that also included cortical and white matter injuries. In the presence of such injuries, children should nevertheless be monitored closely for paroxysmal activity during sleep and cognitive deterioration (Kelemen *et al.*, 2006).

Taken together, the available data support a role for the thalamus in the pathophysiology of ESES and other childhood focal epilepsies, not at the forefront of IED production, but as a necessary facilitator of sleep-related IEDs. This emphasizes the concept of the "cortico-thalamo-cortical loop", which seems to require cortical dysfunction as well as thalamic overexcitation to produce the EEG pattern of ESES (Sánchez Fernández et al., 2013). A change in the regulatory loop, induced by cortical alterations (structural or not), could result in a loss of feed-forward inhibition to thalamocortical neurons and favours a robust oscillatory cortico-thalamo-cortical network (Beenhakker and Huguenard, 2009; Paz et al., 2010). On the other hand, the presence of a cortical deafferentation from thalamic inputs could also alter this loop and create a state of cortical hyperexcitability. The reason why only a percentage of children develop ESES remains unanswered. One hypothesis could be the severity or specificity of cortico-thalamic circuitry damage and/or rearrangements (Halász et al., 2005; Kelemen et al., 2006; Sánchez Fernández et al., 2013). Again, the presence of certain region-specific genetic predispositions such as mutations in the *GRIN2A* gene, might precipitate the appearance of this syndrome (Lemke et al., 2013; Lesca et al., 2013; Turner et al., 2015).

■ Conclusion

Activation of IEDs during NREM sleep is a well-described phenomenon that occurs in the majority of epileptic syndromes. In adults with drug-resistant focal epilepsy, IED activation seems to be related to SWA and arousal fluctuations, especially with phase A1 of the CAP (Ferrillo et al., 2000; Parrino et al., 2006; Ujma et al., 2015). In most childhood focal epileptic syndromes, including ESES, IED activation during sleep seems primarily associated with SFA rather than SWA (Ferrillo et al., 2000b; Nobili et al., 2001). In ESES, however, such an activation is extremely pronounced. The reason for this is still unclear although evidence suggests the necessary interplay between the cortex and the thalamus. Indeed, the role of the thalamus, as part of the "cortico-thalamo-cortical loop", seems essential but not at the forefront of the pathophysiology. Linking the anatomo-electro-clinical findings and the genetic profile with sleep disturbances and cognitive impairment might be key in future studies to elucidate and perhaps halt this harmful developmental process.

Encephalopathy related to Status Epilepticus during slow Sleep: a link with sleep homeostasis?

Guido Rubboli, Reto Huber, Giulio Tononi, Carlo Alberto Tassinari

Sleep is beneficial for cognition by actively participating in learning, language acquisition and memory consolidation. A wealth of experimental data in healthy adults and children have demonstrated the positive effects of post-training sleep in the consolidation of recently learned information (Stickgold et al., 2000; Walker et al., 2002; Fenn et al., 2003; Diekelmann and Born, 2010; Schreiner and Rasch, 2017). These works imply that chronic sleep disturbances in the critical period of brain maturation may have adverse effects on learning and development.

In recent years, a growing body of evidence has suggested that a sleep disruption due to epileptic activity may play a role in the cognitive impairment observed in children suffering from epilepsy (Holmes and Lenck-Santini, 2006; Parisi et al., 2010; Chan et al., 2011; Urbain et al., 2013). Several studies have demonstrated in benign focal epilepsies of childhood as well as in epileptic encephalopathies an association between cognitive and behavioural dysfunctions and the amount of epileptic activity during NREM sleep, supporting the hypothesis that epileptic discharges during NREM sleep can exert negative effects on cognitive abilities (Tassinari and Rubboli, 2006; Massa et al., 2011; Ebus et al., 2011; Van Bogaert et al., 2012; Filippini et al., 2013). Further support to this hypothesis is provided by data showing that improvement of cognitive abilities is strongly correlated with reduction or disappearance of epileptiform discharges during sleep even though normalization of the EEG does not appear to be the only predictive factor (Soprano et al., 1994). Yet, the pathophysiological mechanisms linking the appearance of neuropsychological deficits and epileptic activity during sleep remain largely speculative. Here we review some recent data on a peculiar childhood epileptic syndrome that can represent a model for the investigation of the complex and reciprocal interactions among epileptic activity, sleep physiology and cognitive functions in the developmental age, *i.e.* the "Encephalopathy related to Status Epilepticus during slow Sleep" (ESES) and we discuss how these findings may provide some clues for the understanding of the links between cognitive impairment, sleep disruption, and epileptic activity during NREM sleep.

■ EEG and cognition in ESES

ESES is an age-dependent self-limited epileptic condition characterized by:

– onset in infancy or childhood (with a peak around the age of 4-5 years);

– heterogeneous types of epileptic seizures;

– a typical EEG pattern characterized by continuous or subcontinuous epileptic activity during non REM (NREM) sleep that can last for several months or years;

– variable neuropsychological regression (consisting of IQ decrease, reduction of language), disturbances of behavior (such as development of autistic features, psychotic states), and motor impairment occurring in conjunction with the appearance of the abnormal sleep EEG pattern (Tassinari et al., 2000).

In spite of the favourable long-term prognosis of the epilepsy and of the normalization of the EEG, cognitive deficits and behavioural disorders may persist for life.

A striking feature of ESES is the extreme amount of epileptic discharges occurring during sleep, up to a spike-wave index (SWI) of 85-100% of the time spent in NREM sleep (*figure 1*). This feature led to the eponym of "Electrical Status Epilepticus during Sleep" in the original description by Patry, Lyagoubi and Tassinari (Patry *et al.*, 1971). A few years later, Tassinari *et al.* (1977) reporting an additional series of patients, proposed that the "status epilepticus during sleep" (*i.e.*, SES) was responsible for an encephalopathy characterized primarily by cognitive and behavioural dysfunctions and named it "Encephalopathy related to Status Epilepticus during slow Sleep" (*i.e.* ESES). The SES is thought to have a focal cortical origin that acts as a trigger for the spread of epileptic abnormalities through a secondary bilateral synchrony mechanism (Blume and Pillay, 1985; Kobayashi

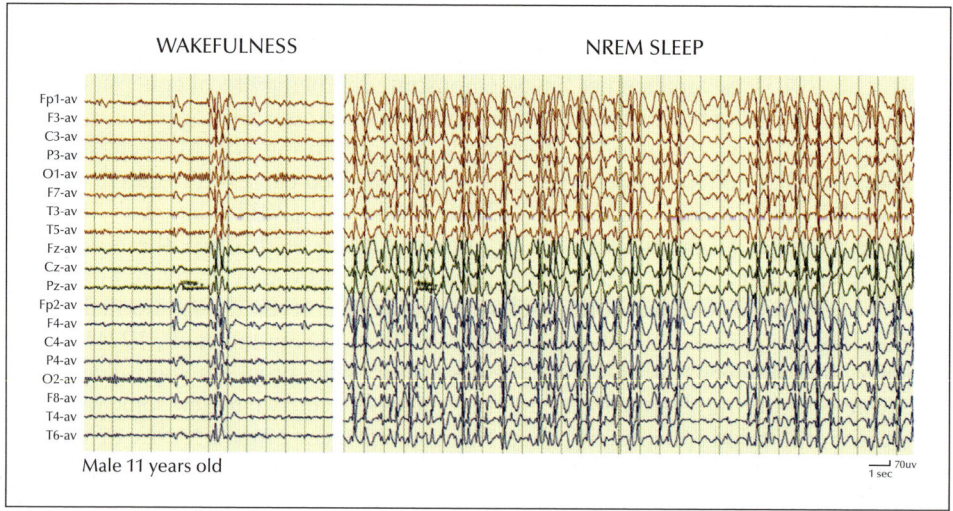

Figure 1/ An eleven-year-old boy suffering from ESES syndrome since the age of eight years. EEG during wakefulness (left) showed normal background activity and sporadic spikes in the right frontal region, sometimes with bifrontal or diffuse spreading. During NREM sleep (right), extreme activation of diffuse spike-and wave discharges that occupied most of NREM sleep was noted (spike-wave index: 87%).

et al., 1994). A focal origin of the epileptic discharges is suggested by the focal nature of the main seizure type, by the observation of focal EEG activity in wakefulness or REM sleep, by intracerebral EEG recordings (Solomon *et al.*, 1993), by the spike phase reversal and interhemispheric peak latencies over unilateral regions (Morikawa *et al.*, 1995), and by focal metabolic abnormalities demonstrated by functional imaging studies (PET, SPECT, fMRI studies) (Hirsch *et al.*, 1990; Mouridsen *et al.*, 1993; Maquet *et al.*, 1995; De Tiège *et al.*, 2009; Siniatchkin *et al.*, 2010). The focal epileptic activity would then engage thalamo-cortical networks underlying the slow oscillations of sleep (Destexhe and Sejnowski, 2001) and enhance their synchrony, promoting their evolution into spike-wave seizures (Amzica and Steriade, 2000) (see also Gibbs *et al.*, p. 54-61). Changes in thalamic firing levels can also switch the cortical dynamics from a desynchronized to a synchronized state and contribute to the synchronization of spike-wave discharges in the cortex (Hirata and Castro-Alamancos, 2010; Liu *et al.*, 2015). These mechanisms may play a role also in the progression and possibly in the maintenance of SES. A role of the thalamus is also supported by evidence of early thalamic injuries in children with ESES (Guzzetta *et al.*, 2005; Sánchez Fernández *et al.*, 2012).

Besides the peculiar sleep EEG pattern, the most intriguing aspect of ESES is the relationship between the onset of SES and the appearance of an encephalopathy accompanied by prominent cognitive and behavioural disturbances, which may persist permanently, or only partially recover, after the resolution of SES and disappearance of seizures (Tassinari *et al.*, 2000, 2019; Seegmüller *et al.*, 2012; Caraballo *et al.*, 2013, see also Arzimanoglou and Cross, p. 77-81, and Dorris *et al.*, p. 83-92). The onset of neuropsychological symptoms follows closely the onset of status epilepticus, and the degree and type of cognitive/behavioural dysfunction seem to depend on the duration and localization of the focal epileptic activity (Tassinari and Rubboli, 2006; Tassinari *et al.*, 2019). These observations have led to the hypothesis that epileptic discharges during sleep may disrupt cognitive and/or motor functions, even when they remain subclinical. Indeed, such epileptic activity (Patry *et al.*, 1971), while originally considered "subclinical" because of the lack of overt electroclinical correlations during sleep, becomes undoubtedly clinical albeit belatedly, due to its effects on cognition and behaviour during wakefulness. These concepts, proposed by Tassinari *et al.* in 1977, have been assimilated into the recent definition of "epileptic encephalopathy" by the International League Against Epilepsy (ILAE) Classification Task Force. This term encompasses not only the conditions with frequent seizures but also those with abundant "interictal" epileptiform abnormalities in which epileptic activities "per se" exert an effect in the development of severe cognitive and behavioural impairments "above and beyond what might be expected from the underlying pathology alone" (Berg *et al.*, 2010).

■ Sleep homeostasis and cognition

What are the pathophysiological mechanisms by which prolonged epileptic activity during sleep leads to the development of the cognitive impairment and behavioural derangement? An intriguing possibility is that the negative effects of ESES may be linked to an excessive engagement of the process of synaptic homeostasis thought to occur during normal sleep (Tassinari and Rubboli, 2006).

Sleep is a homeostatic process: the longer we stay awake, the more intensely we need to sleep, and only sleep can lead to brain restoration after wakefulness (Borbély and

Achermann, 2005). Sleep need is reflected in EEG slow wave activity (SWA, 1-4,5 Hz) during NREM sleep in all mammalian species investigated so far: SWA increases exponentially as a function of prior wakefulness and decreases exponentially during sleep (Tobler, 2000; Borbély and Achermann, 2005). In recent years, a number of studies have shown that sleep homeostasis is closely related to cortical plasticity processes (Tononi and Cirelli, 2014). Specifically, wakefulness, which is typically associated with learning and memory formation, leads to a net increase in synaptic strength and to cellular stress. By contrast, sleep promotes net synaptic depression and renormalization, memory consolidation, and cellular recovery (Vyazovskiy et al., 2008; Maret et al., 2011; Bushey et al., 2011; Tononi and Cirelli, 2014; de Vivo et al., 2017; Diering et al., 2017). Furthermore, both human and animal studies have demonstrated a link between changes in synaptic strength and sleep SWA. A net increase in synaptic strength during wakefulness leads to stronger coupling and therefore increased synchrony among neurons, which is reflected in slow waves of larger amplitude that are steeper during sleep (Esser et al., 2007; Vyazovskiy et al., 2009). On the other hand, slow waves occurring during sleep are thought to promote a progressive down-selection of synapses, which in turn reduces the amplitude of slow waves and, under normal condition, reaches a set point at which SWA is sufficiently low and down-selection stops (*figure 2*). Importantly, the homeostatic regulation of sleep slow waves also has a local component. Learning tasks that produce local strengthening of connections are followed by a local increase in sleep

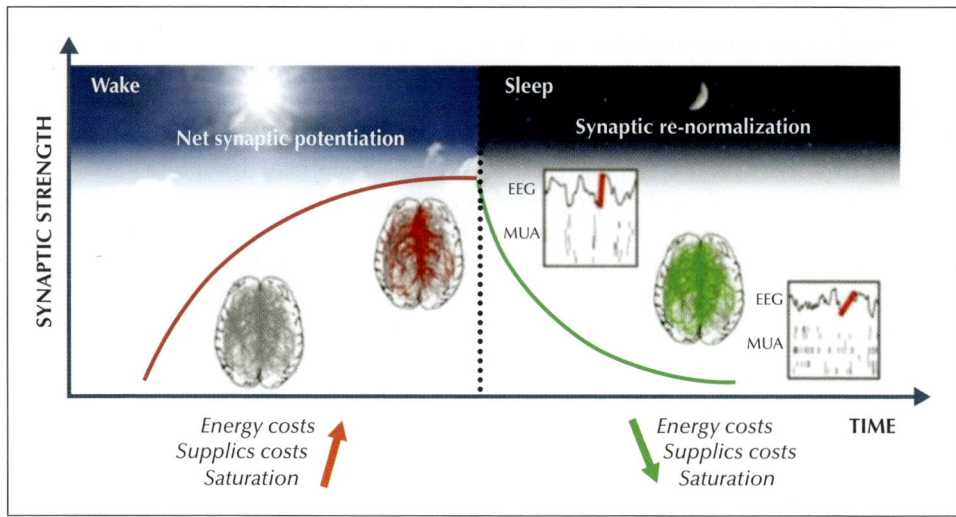

Figure 2/ Summary of the synaptic homeostasis hypothesis: due to learning during the day, wakefulness leads to a net increase in synaptic strength (red line increasing exponentially with time) in select neural circuits (red lines in the schematic of the brain). Wakefulness-related synaptic potentiation is associated with increased need for energy and supplies and saturates the ability of neurons to undergo further potentiation. Sleep at night leads to an overall decrease in synaptic strength (green lines), thus reducing costs at the cellular level (energy, supplies) and at the system level (saturation). At night, the EEG slow waves are large and their slope is steep at the beginning of sleep (early sleep), reflecting higher coupling and synchrony among neurons due to wakefulness-related synaptic potentiation. Multiunit activity (MUA) shows ON and OFF periods occurring highly synchronously across neurons (each row is one neuron and each line is one spike). In late sleep, instead, after synaptic renormalization has occurred, slow waves are smaller and their slope is less steep, because neuronal connections have weakened and neurons no longer undergo ON and OFF states very synchronously.

slow waves (Huber *et al.*, 2004), whereas interventions that lead to non-physiological synaptic depression such as arm immobilization or low frequency TMS are followed by a local decrease in slow wave activity (Huber *et al.*, 2006) (reviewed in Tononi and Cirelli, 2014).

■ Synaptic plasticity and sleep homeostasis

The link between synaptic plasticity and sleep homeostasis is likely to be especially important during development. The architecture of synaptic connections in the cerebral cortex is wired and optimized throughout childhood and adolescence (Rakic *et al.*, 1994). The balancing of synaptic strength across sleep and waking may thus be essential for cortical maturation and thus normal cortical functioning. Intriguingly, sleep slow wave activity peaks during childhood and decreases progressively in the course of adolescence in a way that appears correlated with the occurrence of synaptic refinement in cortical circuits (Huttenlocher, 1979; Feinberg, 1982; Jha *et al.*, 2005; Campbell and Feinberg, 2009; Nelson *et al.*, 2013; Olini *et al.*, 2013; de Vivo *et al.*, 2014; Hoel *et al.*, 2016). Moreover, the topographic distribution of SWA during cortical maturation highlights the developmental changes in cortical plasticity: SWA is highest over posterior regions during early childhood and then shows a spatial shift to anterior regions, reaching the frontal cortex in late adolescence (Kurth *et al.*, 2010). Critically, the maturation of specific skills is predicted by the topographical distribution of SWA, the more frontal the topography of SWA, the better adolescents perform in tasks known to be frontally-mediated (Kurth *et al.*, 2012). Thus, both human and animal studies show a close correspondence between the maturation of the cortex, SWA and behaviour.

■ Impaired synaptic homeostasis in ESES

The occurrence of massive spike wave activity during slow wave sleep every night in children with ESES would be expected to interfere with sleep homeostasis. A sensitive indicator of changes in synaptic strength and associated sleep homeostasis is the slope of sleep slow waves (Esser *et al.*, 2007; Riedner *et al.*, 2007; Vyazovskiy *et al.*, 2007). In healthy control subjects (adults, adolescents and children), the slope of slow waves decreases across sleep (Riedner *et al.*, 2007; Kurth *et al.*, 2010). Children suffering from ESES do not show such a decrease, as if the homeostatic recovery of sleep were impaired (Bolsterli *et al.*, 2011) (*figure 3*). A follow-up study showed that the impairment was most severe at the epileptic focus and that this impairment was positively correlated with the SWI (Bolsterli Heinzle *et al.*, 2014). Moreover, while healthy children showed an increased recall of learned word pairs after a night of sleep, children with ESES showed instead a decrease (Urbain *et al.*, 2011). In one child, hydrocortisone treatment normalized both the sleep EEG and overnight performance (another child whose EEG was only partially improved showed no improvement), suggesting that the impairment of sleep homeostasis may be responsible for the lack of memory consolidation. Finally, Boelsterli *et al.* (2017) have recently shown in children with idiopathic ESES that cognitive/behavioural outcome might correlate with the degree of impairment of the slope of the sleep slow waves. Indeed, complete cognitive/behavioral recovery after ESES was observed in those children in whom the overnight decline of the slope of sleep slow waves during ESES active phase was partially preserved; on the contrary, lack of decline of the slope of sleep slow waves was associated with persistent neuropsychological deficits after ESES resolution. Interestingly, reduced overnight slope

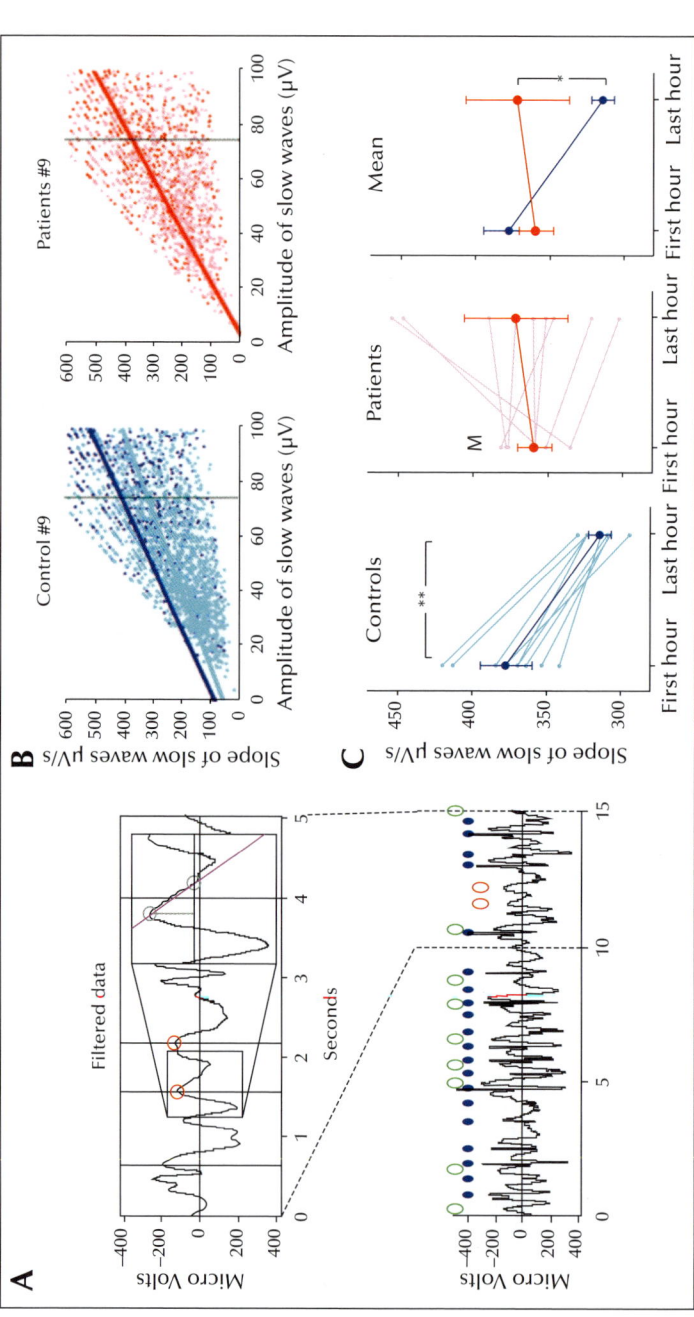

Figure 3/ Impairment of synaptic homeostasis in ESES (adapted from Bolsterli et al., 2011). (A) Slow wave detection method in ESES tracing and extraction of the slope of the slow wave. Below: the tracing reproduces 15 s of the raw signal from one EEG lead during NREM sleep. Circles indicate detected waves, bold red circles indicate waves entering the analysis and bold green circles indicate waves that were excluded because they were part of a spike wave complex (spikes are indicated by small blue dots). Above: 5 s of band-pass filtered signal of the same EEG lead are enlarged. Slow waves identified according to the method proposed by Riedner et al. (2007) are indicated by bold red circles. In the inlet on the right, the extraction of the slope for the first of the two waves is illustrated. The slope was defined as the amplitude of the negative peak divided by the time interval between the negative peak and the following zero crossing (light grey circles). (B) Ascending slope as a function of amplitude in a control subject and in an ESES patient. Scatter plots of the ascending slope of all selected slow waves against their amplitude in the first (blue dots for control, red dots for ESES child) and last hour of sleep (light blue for control, pink for ESES child). For each hour, a regression line was fitted to the data (blue and light blue for the control; red and pink for the ESES patient). Note that in the ESES patient, the line corresponding to the last hour (pink) is hidden behind the red line corresponding to the first hour, indicating no changes in slope between the first and last hour. On the contrary, a shift of the regression line across the night is observed in the control subject. The vertical black line indicates the voltage (75 uV) at which the ascending slopes were compared between the first and last hour. (C) Changes of the slope of slow waves during the night. Ascending slopes at an amplitude of 75 uV in the first and last hour of sleep are shown for control subjects (left) and patients (middle). Solid lines indicate the group mean. Error bars illustrate s.e.m. In the right panel, the superimposition of the mean slope (± s.e.m.) of control subjects (blue line) and patients (red line) shows that the slope of slow waves did not differ between patients and control subjects in the first hour of sleep, but was significantly steeper in patients compared to control subjects in the last hour of sleep, suggesting an impairment of the homeostatic recovery of sleep in ESES (**$p<0.001$, paired t-test; *$p<0.01$, unpaired t-test).

decline of sleep slow waves has been shown to be related to poorer learning during wakefulness also in adult patients with focal epilepsy (Boly et al., 2017).

■ Spikes, synaptic homeostasis and cognition

If normal sleep plays a fundamental role in synaptic renormalization, it is natural to ask whether epileptic activity during NREM sleep may interfere with the homeostatic renormalization of synapses and produce instead abnormal synaptic potentiation. Such abnormal plasticity, recurring nightly for months and years, might eventually lead to a severe impairment of the cognitive functions and behaviour mediated by the affected brain areas (Buzsaki, 1998; Tassinari and Rubboli, 2006; Romcy-Pereira et al., 2009). In animal models, epileptic discharges occurring during wakefulness lead to long-term synaptic potentiation (LTP) (Buzsáki, 1989; Leite et al., 2005; Romcy-Pereira et al., 2009) by hijacking the mechanisms of learning in a maladaptive manner, unrelated to environmental inputs. It is likely that epileptic discharges occurring during sleep also induce plastic changes, although it is unclear in which direction: potentiation, as is normally the case in wakefulness, or depression, as is normally the case in NREM sleep.

The SWA of NREM results from an ongoing alternation between a depolarized 'up-state', when neurons fire tonically, and a hyperpolarized 'down-state', when neurons stop firing for hundreds of milliseconds (Amzica and Steriade, 1998). Laminar recordings of local field potentials, and of multiple- and single-unit activities during intracerebral recordings in humans have shown that the 'up-state' of sleep slow waves is associated with multi-unit-activity bursts as well as high-frequency oscillations (HFO) (Csercsa et al., 2010; Nir et al., 2011). In cortical areas heavily involved in learning processes, SWA, slow wave slopes, and the synchrony of HFO during the "up-state" increase together. Intriguingly, a recent study in ESES has demonstrated the occurrence of exaggerated HFO related to epileptic spikes (Kobayashi et al., 2010). Such pathological HFO occurring systematically throughout NREM sleep are likely to produce major abnormalities in synaptic plasticity and impair the synaptic renormalization processes.

Such an impairment would be especially harmful during the critical period of cortical maturation in childhood and pre-adolescence, which is characterized by massive synaptogenesis, synaptic pruning, and the refinement of synaptic circuits (Huttenlocher, 1979; Huttenlocher and Dabholkar, 1997; Petanjek et al., 2011; Liu et al., 2012). In this critical period, plastic changes involve all cortical laminae and thalamo-cortical inputs (Issa, 2014) and local increases of learning-related SWA are strongest (Wilhelm et al., 2014). It is well-established that the maturation of cortical circuits during adolescence occurs in parallel with a progressive reduction of SWA (Buchmann et al., 2011; Campbell et al., 2011). Recently, computer simulations have shown that this developmental decline of SWA can track activity-dependent synaptic refinement that underlies the proper functioning of neural circuits (Hoel et al., 2016). In animal models, interfering with cortical activity during NREM sleep leads to a deterioration of previously acquired cortical adaptations (Frank et al., 2001). Altogether, these data suggest that a systematic impairment of synaptic renormalization during NREM sleep would lead to profound, possibly irreversible changes in cortical wiring, which may thus represent an unfortunate consequence of "subclinical" epileptic activity in the active phase of ESES. Such a model would provide an explanation for the loss of acquired functions, such as language, and for the persistence of cognitive and behavioural disturbances after the end of ESES. The report of prefrontal lobe growth during the active phase in a patient with ESES may also be a macroscopic anatomical consequence of impaired synaptic renormalization during sleep (Kanemura et al., 2009).

In summary, an impairment of synaptic renormalization due to epileptic activity during NREM sleep could explain many of the clinical features in children with ESES, and possibly in other forms of childhood epilepsy with a striking increment of paroxysmal abnormalities during NREM sleep or with altered slow wave activity (e.g. West syndrome patients; Fattinger et al., 2015). The clinical implication is that such "subclinical" abnormalities during critical developmental periods should be seriously considered, as they may alter cortical wiring and thereby disrupt cognitive and behavioural functions irreversibly. Future studies should explore whether in epileptic children with high SWI during sleep and absent or minor cognitive disturbances, the reduction of the slope of the slow waves during sleep is preserved or minimally affected, reflecting a preservation or minimal perturbance of synaptic renormalization. This realization calls for careful testing, including neuropsychological and behavioural tools to detect selective or subtle cognitive dysfunctions related to a highly focal ESES (Kuki et al., 2014), that coupled with sophisticated neuroimaging, and the use of novel EEG indices, in addition to SWI, such as the decline of slow wave slopes in NREM sleep, might be useful for a timely diagnosis and treatment, and might provide indirect information on the cortical networks underlying specific cognitive functions (Tassinari et al., 2015).

Cognitive impairment and behavioral disorders in Encephalopathy related to Status Epilepticus during slow Sleep: diagnostic assessment and outcome

Alexis Arzimanoglou, Helen J. Cross

Studies describing quantitative aspects of epileptiform abnormalities on EEG are overrepresented in the literature, whereas those evaluating evolution of cognition and behavior are undervalued. The large variation in the design of the studies, the tests used, the age ranges evaluated and the variability in outcome measures preclude any reasonable comparison. Consequently, studies attributing improvement exclusively to epileptiform discharges should be interpreted with caution (Sanchez Fernandez *et al.*, 2015). Probably the only relatively strong data available suggests that severity and duration of initial regression are the most important risk factors of cognitive impairment in the long term (Van Bogaert, 2013).

■ Outcome and predictors of outcome

Electrical status epilepticus of slow sleep is by definition what could be classified as a true epileptic encephalopathy. It is believed that cognitive and behavioural difficulties are the direct result of the underlying epileptic activity and any targeted treatments. However, we need to review the evidence on outcome; specifically, the relationship with resolution of the epileptiform activity, the influence of aetiology and indeed the role of treatment. Further, do we have evidence that we can actually influence outcome?

Like other epilepsy syndromes, Encephalopathy related to Status Epilepticus during slow Sleep (ESES) is described on the basis of electroclinical features but may have many aetiologies - specifically lesional and non-lesional. Presentation of cognitive deficit has been suggested to be related to the geographical prominence of spike wave activity - in Landau-Kleffner, this is seen with temporal prominence, whereas more global problems are associated with a frontocentral focus. However, there does not appear to be any evidence of a predictor of outcome dependent on localisation of epileptiform discharges.

Many have demonstrated ESES to be an age-related phenomenon; illustrated by both lesional and nonlesional cases. It has been well demonstrated that children with *hemipolymicrogyria* may present with focal seizures but can subsequently evolve with development of atonic attacks associated with the finding of electrical status epilepticus of slow sleep. In longitudinal studies, such attacks resolve along with the ESES (Guerrini et al., 1998; Caraballo et al., 2013) - however, there are no cognitive or behaviour measures included in the studies reported, so the overall impact on this aspect is unknown. It is now known that such phenomena occur in "acquired" cases or those with developmental pathology and may occur with unilateral or bilateral disease. In the case of unilateral structural abnormalities, surgery has been demonstrated to resolve the ESES but definitive improved cognitive outcome, although suspected as being likely, has not been proven (Loddenkemper et al., 2009).

There are many methodological problems with long-term studies reported to date within the literature. Not least, series often include both lesional and non-esional cases, with very small numbers owing to the rarity of the condition. Further, there is significant heterogeneity in the treatment utilised even in a single centre with no structured protocols, which applies also to reporting of outcome and time period (van den Munckhof et al., 2015). The natural history is such that electrical status epilepticus has a good prognosis and resolves with age - it is difficult to know therefore the impact of any intervention over time. This is well illustrated by the surgical Landau Kleffner series of Morrell; the initial series of 14/54 children who underwent surgery (multiple subpial transection) after full assessment although 6 had normal speech postoperatively and five improved (Morrell et al., 1995; Grote et al., 1999); a later follow-up study demonstrated that the extent of improvement was related to time from surgery. Indeed, a recently reported study showed no difference in outcome as to whether surgery was undertaken or not (Downes et al., 2015).

Praline et al., (2003) reported on seven adults who had experienced CSWS or Landau Kleffner Syndrome in childhood. At the time of review, they were aged 16-26 years; five had CSWS syndrome and two Landau Kleffner. They confirmed the epilepsy to have a good prognosis in the long-term; only one had continuing active epilepsy. However, 3/5 who had CSWS in childhood remained significantly cognitively impaired (Praline et al., 2003).

Possible predictors of outcome include age at onset, duration of ESES, response to treatment, aetiology and predominant location of the interictal focus. An older age at onset and shorter duration of ESES are correlated with a better cognitive outcome although this does not appear to be absolute (Scholtes et al., 2005). This aside, in a further study of 10 patients with non-lesional ESES followed for 15.6 years, patients with prolonged global intellectual regression had the worst outcome whereas those with more specific and short-lived deficits showed the best recovery (Seegmuller et al., 2012). Further, there was no correlation between outcome an age at onset or age at cessation of ESES, but the three most severely affected individuals had the longest duration of ESES. Kramer et al. reported on 30 patients from four clinics who had been determined to have ESES; 20 had an associated intellectual regression, having previously been normal, 3 of whom did not respond to treatment. They found a significant correlation between residual cognitive deficits and the total ESES period (Kramer et al., 2009). However, careful longitudinal review has illustrated that although such correlations are evident, prognosis of an individual is highly variable.

Pera et al. (2013) reviewed 25 children with a mean follow-up of 13.5 years; they suggested five patterns of clinical course within this otherwise small series with not necessarily a

Table 1. Minimum technical requirements for polygraphic recordings of ESES/CSWS*

1. For the diagnosis at least one overnight polygraphic recording is required.
2. For follow-up an overnight sleep recording is recommended, however a nap polygraphy can be sufficient.
3. In both cases (overnight and nap polygraphy), it is mandatory: • to acquire both wakefulness and sleep in the same recording; • to assess sleep stages, thus it is essential to acquire both EEG and polygraphic signals (see below).
4. All signals should be digitized and stored with sampling rates at least of 250 Hz (higher sampling rates – 512, 1024 Hz or superior – are strongly encouraged).
5. EEG: • at least 19 electrodes should be used, based on the 10-20 system (Fp1, Fp2, F7, F3, Fz, F4, F8, T3, C3, Cz, C4, T4, T5, P3, Pz, P4, T6, O1, O2). The use of higher number of electrodes (i.e. 10-10 system) or supernumerary electrodes is encouraged; • digital recording reference should be an additional electrode (or combination of electrodes), and not one of those in the 10-10 or 10-20 system. Additional electrodes at POz and Fpz are frequently used as 'common reference' and 'subject ground', respectively.
6. Electroculogram (EOG): • at least two bipolar EOG channels should be included. The recommended procedure is to place one electrode approximately 1 cm above and slightly lateral to the outer canthus of right eye (right-EOG or ROC) and another electrode 1 cm below and slightly lateral to the outer canthus of the left eye (left-EOG or LOC), both referred to the same (right) ear or mastoid electrode (alternatively each ROC and LOC could be referred to the respective contralateral mastoid).
7. Electromyograms (EMG): • one antigravitary muscle (either mylohyoideus or submentalis or mentalis muscle); • one limb muscle (either leg – i.e. tibialis anterior – or arm – i.e. extensor digitorum – muscle).
8. Pneumogram (PNG): • at least one belt – equipped with piezoelectric or inductance-plethysmography sensors – placed around the thoracic or abdominal compartments to measure the tension changes as a surrogate for measuring respiratory effort.
9. Electrocardiogram

(*) Prepared in collaboration with G. Rubboli and G. Cantalupo.

clear correlation between clinical course and EEG response to treatment. Group 1 demonstrated the classical regression with EEG abnormality, and improvement with EEG response to treatment; Group 2 had predominantly motor deficit with minimal cognitive change; Group 3 had cognitive deficits that persisted despite improvement in the EEG; Group 4 had associated cerebral lesions, with little change in cognition over time; and Group 5 included two patients with progressive deterioration based on neuropsychological tests without temporal correlation with ESES duration (less than seven months), and no association with clinical and electroencephalographic relapses. In total, 44% of the whole group had permanent cognitive impairment in the long term (Pera et al., 2013).

■ Diagnostic assessment of cognition and behavior in ESES

Because ESES is a highly heterogeneous and a relatively rare entity (even when atypical forms are included), multicentric studies usually fail in reaching a statistically significant number of participants; long-term follow-up is usually not possible, often because of lack of funding. However, improving our knowledge on outcome requires a method to measure it.

Lessons from the past should lead the epileptological community to a more pragmatic approach and avoidance of circular statements; instead of indefinitely concluding that *"controlled multicentric studies are needed..."* we could agree upon a basic diagnostic assessment protocol to be followed by all major paediatric epilepsy centers.

A common-to-all, basic diagnostic assessment protocol

All children with ESES, independent of underlying etiology, should **from onset** be referred to a pediatric neurology center specialized in epilepsy. A commonly agreed, user-friendly software could be used to collect relevant data (that one day, if needed, could be merged into a common database) to include:

- main neurological and somatic examination findings at onset;
- family history, including familial cognitive and behavioral problems;
- a minimum 24-hour video-EEG, preferably before administration of any treatment or within the first 8 weeks; agreement could be made upon a set of minimum technical requirements for polygraphic recordings (*table 1*);
- the realization of a predefined, commonly agreed, core battery of neurocognitive tests and evaluation scales (see below) covering the most crucial parameters, sufficiently straightforward to be reproduced in different clinical settings;
- high-resolution MRI performed according to standard epilepsy protocols (Gaillard et al., 2009);
- genetic evaluation (to be enriched on the basis of progress made in the field).

Practices that may need a consensual attitude

- An agreement on the first three AEDs to be used, including dose per kg, duration of each trial and minimal efficacy criteria. Lack of results from controlled trials should oblige us all to follow a consensual approach, referring to existing open studies, rather than a dogmatic position based on personal beliefs and impressions;
- An agreement upon a core battery of neurocognitive tests, to be repeated at regular intervals (once a year?). Depending on the ages and abilities of the patients, tests should cover the major domains of cognition (intelligence, language, memory, attention, visuospatial functions, executive functions);
- An agreement upon a basic scale evaluating AED side effects (Morita et al., 2012) to be repeated at regular intervals, particularly after a change in AED therapy; This could be systematically coupled to a sensitive and time-efficient screening tool for attention and executive functions, such as EpiTrack Junior (Kadish et al., 2013).

Practices that probably can only be decided arbitrarily !

An agreement upon intervals for 24H VEEG. Variability in current practices complicates comparison of findings across various studies, and limits the possibility of generating evidence-based guidelines for patient follow-up (Jehi et al., 2015). The reason that such an agreement between centres is hard to obtain probably reflects a disagreement upon primary efficacy criteria. One, rather classical, approach would be the "percentage of amelioration of the sleep-EEG ESES pattern", reproducing what we are currently applying in the majority of centres.

However, another option, probably better serving our primary aim (see above) could be to use the results from core battery neuropsychological tests as an efficacy criterion. For example, at least for a period of 12 months, the AED prescribed would be replaced only in case of signs of cognitive deterioration (validated by a minimum of tests) or in case of clinically identifiable epileptic seizures. EEG variations would still be recorded without automatically leading to modifications of treatment.

If an agreement on the second option suggested above proves impossible to attend, we could at least agree that each individual centre would accept to systematically determine its treatment attitudes on the basis of the same criterion: either EEG variations or the results of the neuropsychological follow-up. Such an approach would at least allow the constitution of two comparable groups, in terms of global evolution in the long-run, of children treated for ESES.

In summary, the fluctuating clinical and EEG courses of ESES complicate the diagnostic process and evaluation of treatment. We need to validate a feasible screening method to be used by clinicians of all major paediatric epilepsy centres. It should be in accordance with the main lines of current clinical practices and preferably under the authority of a well-defined endorsed Task Force such as within the ILAE. The policy of publishing small series of patients per centre has clearly failed in reaching meaningful clinical conclusions. The natural course of the disorder(s) remains poorly known and multiple underlying mechanisms link the EEG patterns to developmental outcomes. A consensus on a homogeneous approach should be considered a priority.

Progressive intellectual impairment in children with Encephalopathy related to Status Epilepticus during slow Sleep

Liam Dorris, Mary O'Regan, Margaret Wilson, Sameer M. Zuberi

Encephalopathy related to Status Epilepticus during slow Sleep or ESES is an age-dependent and self-limited syndrome whose distinctive features include a characteristic age at onset (with a peak around 4-5 years), heterogeneous seizure types (mostly focal motor or unilateral seizures during sleep and absences or falls while awake), a typical EEG pattern (with continuous and diffuse paroxysms occupying a significant proportion of slow wave sleep) and a variable neuropsychological regression consisting of IQ decrease, reduction of language (as in acquired aphasia or Landau-Kleffner syndrome), disturbance of behaviour and motor impairment (in the form of ataxia, dyspraxia, dystonia or unilateral deficit) (Tassinari et al., 2000). The favourable seizure outcome is independent of the etiology and is observed also in cases with cortical malformations such as multilobar polymicrogyria (Guerrini et al 1998). The characteristic EEG patterns during slow wave sleep also disappear at approximately the same time, but focal interictal spikes may persist (Morikawa et al., 1989; Bureau, 1995).

The first description of sub-clinical electrical status induced by sleep in children dates back to 1971 when Patry, Lyagoubi and Tassinari described in six children a peculiar EEG pattern occurring almost continuously in sleep, characterized by apparently 'subclinical' spike and wave for a variable length of time. Tassinari introduced the term "Electrical status epilepticus during slow sleep" and this was originally defined as status epilepticus occurring during at least 85% of slow sleep (Tassinari et al., 1977). More recently, the proportion of affected slow sleep required to affect cognition and behaviour has been recognised to be lower, with some authors suggesting that => 50% can be associated with cognitive sequelae. The most typical paroxysmal discharges on EEG are spike wave at 1.5 to 3.5-Hz polyspikes and polyspikes and wave. Secondary bilateral synchrony is the mechanism underlying continuous spikes and waves during slow sleep. In this respect, the apparently generalized seizures (absences, tonic-clonic seizures) occurring in this condition have, in fact, a focal onset (Tassinari, 1995). ESES can be present at various evolutionary stages within a spectrum of diseases, the prototypes of which are continuous spike and wave in slow sleep (CSWS), Landau Kleffner Syndrome (LKS) and some patients initially presenting with childhood (benign or rolandic) epilepsy with centrotemporal spikes (BECTS) (Galanopolou et al., 2000). Children with ESES generally demonstrate a global neuropsychological disturbance whereas those diagnosed with LKS typically display an isolated language disorder. In both syndromes, recovery of language functions may be associated with disappearance of continuous spike and slow wave during slow wave sleep. The neuropsychological disturbances are suspected to be a function of the genetic or symptomatic origin of the underlying epileptic condition, the cortical area of the primary focal paroxysmal activity, the patient's age and the severity and duration of the EEG abnormalities (De Negri, 1997).

ESES is a rare disorder although accurate incidence is difficult to determine. Morikawa et al found an incidence of 0.5% among 12,854 children evaluated during a 10-year period (Morikawa et al., 1995). The Landau-Kleffner syndrome (LKS) and Encephalopathy related to Status Epilepticus during slow Sleep (ESES) are rare childhood-onset epileptic encephalopathies in which loss of language skills occurs in the context of an epileptiform EEG activated in sleep. Although in LKS the loss of function is limited to language, in ESES there is a wider spectrum of cognitive impairment. The two syndromes are distinct but have some overlap. Whether ESES as a whole should be defined as an independent syndrome or as an electroclinical feature of many epilepsy syndromes is a source of debate (see Hirsch et al., p. 7-16). The duration of electrical status epilepticus during slow sleep has been correlated with the final neuropsychological outcome (Rousselle & Revol, 1995). It has also been suggested that electrical status epilepticus during slow sleep is a model for prolonged cognitive impairment induced by interictal paroxysmal activity (Tassinari, 1995; see also Tassinari and Rubboli, p. 99-103). "Interictal paroxysmal activity" may interfere with different cognitive processes, as demonstrated by neurophysiological, neuropsychological, and biochemical studies (Binnie, 1993; Wasterlain et al., 1993). It has been suggested that interictal epileptiform discharges have a role to play in the language regression seen in some children with autism, however, other studies have contradicted this view (Ballaban-Gil et al., 1998; De Menezes et al., 1998; Goldberg et al., 1998). What is certain from genetic studies is that autism, ESES and epilepsy may share the same underlying aetiologies (Lesca et al., 2012; Wolff et al., 2017).

Following resolution of ESES, improvement in language dysfunction, learning disability and psychiatric disturbances generally occurs but this is variable and individualized. The majority of affected children never return to normal levels, particularly for verbal and attention abilities (Morikawa et al., 1985; Roulet Perez et al., 1993; see also Arzimanoglou and Cross, p. 77-81). Margari et al followed 25 patients (19 male) from 2 to 16 years of age (mean age: 6 years±3 SD) to examine the presence and course of neuropsychiatric disorder (mean duration of follow-up: 3.9 years) (Margari et al., 2012). At diagnosis of CSWS, 54% of patients had behavioral problems, 37.5% mental retardation, 33% learning disabilities, 17% developmental coordination disorder, 12.5% language disorder, and 8% pervasive developmental disorder. During the follow-up, neuropsychiatric dysfunctions remained unaltered in 52% of the patients, worsened in 24%, and improved in only 24%. The authors suggest that CSWS may be associated with a broad spectrum of neuropsychiatric disorders and may promote their worsening over time. Despite the apparent developmental impact of the ESES, there has been very little published related to neuropsychological outcomes, with only two very small cohort studies, e.g. Seegmüller et al. (2012) n=10 patients, and Scholtz et al (2005) n=7 patients.

The current study aimed to provide data on a larger series of children with treated ESES using standardised neuropsychological tests. We aimed to provide some preliminary data on the impact of ESES on the developing brain in terms of intellectual development in middle to late childhood.

■ Methods

Participants were identified by reviewing reports of 24-hour ambulatory EEG over a period of five years (n=2200). The recordings of those who exhibited marked sleep accentuation of epileptiform activity were reviewed. Those who fulfilled the diagnostic criteria for ESES, i.e. >85%, were identified. We also included children who had abnormal activity occupying 60-85% of slow wave sleep if there was a history of change in behavior and/or recent loss of skills. Children who were in non-convulsive status with a continuous dysrhythmia, awake and asleep, were excluded. Clinical records were reviewed to determine seizure types, aetiology, and behavioural and EEG features.

This was a retrospective study with cases managed by several clinicians and no uniform or standardized therapeutic paradigm for ESES. Cases were treated with several different anti-epileptic drugs including clobazam, prednisolone and valproate with variability in dose and combination of different treatments. In addition, the sequence and duration of different therapies was not controlled therefore the data on medication use in individual cases is not presented as no valid conclusions can be drawn from this data.

■ Participants

Twenty-two participants met inclusion criteria (13 males and nine females). The median age of the sample at initial assessment was 6 years (mean: 6.8, sd 2.9 years) with a range of 4-16 years. At follow-up, the median age was 7.5 years (mean: 9.3, sd 3.4 years) with a range of 6-19 years. This created a mean latency period between assessments of 2.5 years. The clinical histories of all patients are described in *table 1*. Thirteen participants were reassessed within three years and eight participants within 3-5 years. Five of 22 had a significant neonatal history and 5/22 had abnormal imaging using MRI/CT. There were heterogenous epilepsy types (*see table 1*).

■ Measures

Participants were assessed using the WISC-III (Wechsler Intelligence Scale for children, version 3, UK norm, UK-edition) or the WPPSI-R (Wechsler Primary and Preschool Scale of Intelligence, revised, UK-edition). When patients were unable to complete all subtests of the WISC/WPPSI, pro-rated scores were derived using statistical techniques outlined within the manual. As this was a retrospective study there was no specified time period between the first and subsequent neuropsychological evaluations.

■ Results

At the time of their initial assessment, nine participants had a measured IQ within the learning disability range, four within the severe range (IQ: 40-49) and five within the mild to moderate range (IQ: 50-69). Four participants had an IQ within the borderline range

Table 1/ Clinical history showing IQ, seizure type, age of onset, imaging and other clinical phenomena for each participant.

Patient	IQ 1	IQ 2	Neonatal history	Developmental history	Age of onset	Type of epilepsy	Age at diagnosis of ESES	Clinical presentation at diagnosis	Maximum epileptic activity	Imaging
1	77	65	Uneventful	Febrile seizure aged 2.5 years	2.5 years	Generalised and focal epilepsy of unknown aetiology	3 years	No cognitive / behavioural concern	Right hemisphere emphasis	CT normal
2	77	68	Uneventful	Normal; mild dyspraxia	4 years	Atypical childhood epilepsy with centrotemporal Spikes	5 years	Language difficulties	Assymetrical ESES, right hemisphere emphasis	CT normal
3	89	56	Hydrocephalus secondary to aqueduct stenosis	VP shunted 2 months; Right hemi paresis; Global cognitive delay	4 years	Focal epilepsy with structural aetiology	8 years	Language and social communication difficulties	Left hemisphere	CT Left sided peri-ventricular white matter loss; PVL
4	40	69	Uneventful	Uneventful	6 years	Focal epilepsy with unknown aetiology	6 years	Language and social communication difficulties	Left hemisphere emphasis (temporal)	MRI normal
5	105	78	Uneventful	Normal	>1 year	Generalised epilepsy with myoclonic seizures (unknown aetiology)	4 years	No cognitive regression noted	Bilateral	MRI normal

Patient	IQ 1	IQ 2	Neonatal history	Developmental history	Age of onset	Type of epilepsy	Age at diagnosis of ESES	Clinical presentation at diagnosis	Maximum epileptic activity	Imaging
6	98	99	Uneventful	Delayed motor development	7 months	Focal epilepsy with unknown aetiology	5 years	Poor educational progress	Bilateral	MRI normal
7	108	108	Premature 26 weeks gestation,	Acquired brain injury aged 7 years,	10 years	Generalised and focal epilepsy with structural aetiology	11 years	Memory and learning problems	Left hemisphere emphasis (temporal)	MRI normal
8	40	40	Uneventful	Global developmental delay, behaviour problems	5 years	Generalised and focal epilepsy of unknown aetiology	5 years	Severe ongoing behavioural problems	bilateral	MRI normal
9	40	40	Uneventful	Global developmental delay	4 years	Focal epilepsy of unknown aetiology	10 years	Increasing concern over poor language and learning	Left emphasis	MRI showed corpus-callosum abnormality
10	81	75	Uneventful	Restricted interests, rigid behaviour	3 years	Focal epilepsy of unknown aetiology	8 years	Continuing concerns	Right sided ESES	MRI abnormal, right-sided peri-ventricular leukomalacia
11	81	75	Uneventful	Specific learning difficulties/ clumsy	6 years	Focal epilepsy of unknown aetiology	6 years	Educational difficulties	Bilateral	MRI normal
12	65	50	Uneventful	Global developmental delay	5 years	Focal epilepsy of unknown aetiology	6 years	Continuing developmental concerns	Bilateral	MRI normal

Patient	IQ 1	IQ 2	Neonatal history	Developmental history	Age of onset	Type of epilepsy	Age at diagnosis of ESES	Clinical presentation at diagnosis	Maximum epileptic activity	Imaging
13	79	62	Neonatal seizures	Mild right hemiplegia;	1st week of life	Focal epilepsy with structural aetiology	7 years	Reduced concentration and deterioration in memory/ reading	Left sided (occipital) ESES	MRI hemi-megalencephaly
14	59	56	Premature 32/40, severe IUGR,	Whooping cough aged 2 years 5 months	Aged 5.5 years	Childhood epilepsy with centrotemporal spikes	7 years	Language difficulties, poor educational progress	Bilateral	None
15	69	69	Neonatal seizures	Left hemiplegia, learning disabilities	15 years	Focal Epilepsy with structural aetiology	15.5 years	Deterioration in school work	Bilateral with Right hemisphere emphasis	MRI right schizencephaly
16	78	69	Uneventful	Normal	3 years	Myoclonic atonic epilepsy	3 years	Behavioural, motor and cognitive regression	Bilateral	MRI normal
17	82	88	Uneventful	Delayed speech and language development	3 years	Focal epilepsy with unknown aetiology	3 years	Continuing speech delay	Bilateral with shifting emphasis	MRI normal
18	40	40	Uneventful	Mutism aged 4 years, normal speech development prior	Aged 4	Landau kleffner syndrome	4 years	Continuing aphasia	Focal ESES left hemisphere	MRI normal

Patient	IQ 1	IQ 2	Neonatal history	Developmental history	Age of onset	Type of epilepsy	Age at diagnosis of ESES	Clinical presentation at diagnosis	Maximum epileptic activity	Imaging
19	106	92	Uneventful	None	5 years	Myoclonic Atonic Epilepsy	5.5 years	Concentration, school difficulties	Bilateral	MRI normal
20	82	70	Uneventful	Normal development	3 years	Focal epilepsy with unknown aetiology	8 years	Concentration, school difficulties	Bilateral	None
21	65	69	Uneventful	Mild learning difficulties, late childhood diagnosis of Tourettes Syndrome treated with haloperidol	11 years	Focal epilepsy with unknown aetiology	12 years	Continuing concentration problems	Right sided ESES	MRI normal
22	110	105	Uneventful	Accidental asphyxia aged 5yrs associated with status epilepticus	2.5 years	Focal epilepsy with structural aetiology	6.5 years	Memory and learning	Bilateral with right sided emphasis	MRI normal

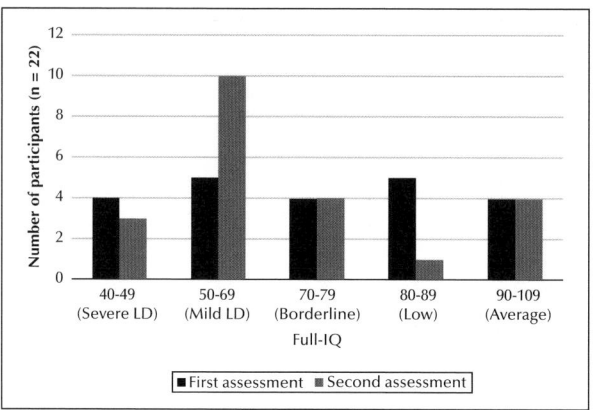

Figure 1/ Intellectual ability levels at first and second assessment (mean time interval 2.5 years).

(IQ: 70-79), five had an IQ within the low-average range (80-89), and a further four had an IQ within the average range (90-109). At follow-up assessment, thirteen participants had measured IQs within the LD range, three within the severe range, and ten within the mild to moderate range. Four participants had an IQ within the borderline range, one within low-average, and four within the average range. Therefore, 41% of the sample had a measured IQ within the learning disability range at first assessment compared to 55% at second assessment; an increase of 14% (*figure 1*).

As the data were not normally distributed, a repeated-measures non-parametric analysis (Wilcoxon) was used to compare group median FSIQ, VIQ and PIQ between assessment points (*figure 2*). There were significant differences in Full-Scale IQ with a small effect size

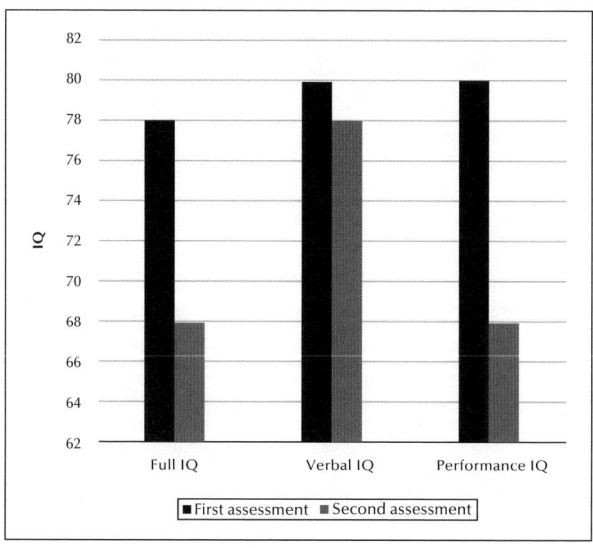

Figure 2/ Changes in cohort median Full IQ, Verbal IQ and Performance IQ between first and second assessments.

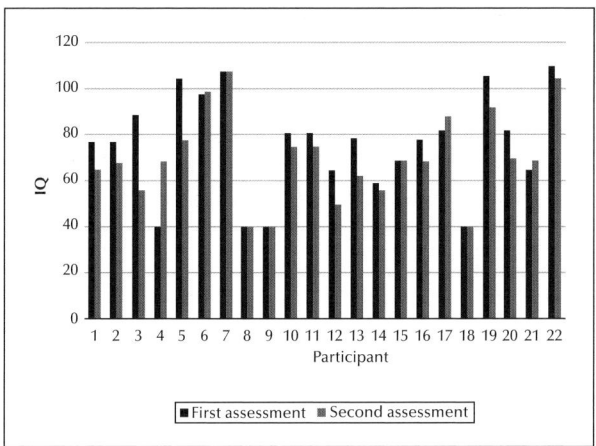

Figure 3/ Individual participant changes in IQ between first and second assessment.

(p=0.042; d=0.3), and performance IQ with a medium effect size (p=0.031; d=0.4). There was no significant difference in VIQ across time (p=0.421).

Figure 3 shows the change in IQ for each participant which can be correlated with the clinical histories shown in *table 1* (the participants 1-22 in table 1 correspond to those in *figure 3*).

To address the important issue of statistical versus clinical significance regarding change in IQ scores, we analyzed the data using a conservative criterion of a =>12-point difference in IQ. When adopting this more conservative criterion to denote clinically significant change, seven participants were found to show a =>12-IQ point change with a mean FSIQ at initial assessment of 86 (sd=15), and at follow-up of 67 (sd=14.7) with a large effect size (d=1.3). The largest effect was observed in Performance IQ with a mean reduction of 24 points from 92 to 68 (p=0.018; d=1.5). A less dramatic drop in VIQ was observed with an average of a 9 point-change (d=0.4). If excluding those participants who scored at floor value at both time points (n=4), our findings suggest that 7/18 participants (38%) showed a highly significant intellectual decline affecting FSIQ and PIQ. These individuals tended to move from the average range to the mild learning disability range. Four individuals had IQ values =<40 (floor value on WISC-III) at both assessments and therefore were not able to be rated in terms of on-going cognitive loss using these instruments.

■ Discussion

We report the largest neuropsychological outcome study of childhood ESES with main findings of a clinically and statistically significant decrease in Full-Scale and Performance IQ despite treatment. Around one-third (7/22) of participants in the current study showed a highly significant loss (=>12pts) in intellectual performance, evident particularly within their Performance IQ scores within a relatively short period of time (2.5 years). These individuals tended to move from the average range to the mild learning disability range and were not distinguishable from the rest of the sample in terms of clinical history, imaging or duration of ESES. Performance IQ (PIQ) effects were more pronounced than for verbal

IQ, a finding of interest as language difficulties are the most commonly reported difficulties in these children, and may reflect reduced processing speed, working memory and overall cognitive efficiency.

Whilst there have been several descriptions of the clinical and behavioural manifestations of ESES, few have used standardized tests to look at cognitive function. In a report of longitudinal neuropsychological outcome in 10 patients followed from the time of diagnosis into adulthood (mean follow-up duration of 15.6 years), six patients had an IQ <70, two had a low IQ (77 and 84), and two had an IQ within the average range (103 and 85) (Seegmuller et al., 2012). The authors also describe social, cognitive and attention difficulties in the majority of the patients. They suggest that the initial severity and duration of the acute phase regression and the duration of ESES were most predictive of poorer neuropsychological outcome. In another report it was suggested that the initial diagnosis had little prognostic significance, but that length and the age at onset of CSWS, the site of epileptiform activity and the individual neuropsychological profile are more useful for predictors of long-term cognitive outcome (Veggiotti, 2012).

Our study has limitations as a result of the retrospective nature and lack of control over timing of assessments and therapeutic interventions. We relied on a single outcome measure, i.e. IQ testing, and whilst the predictive utility, validity and reliability of standardized IQ tests are high (Dorris et al., 2017), it would be useful for future studies to include measures of adaptive behavior, Quality of Life and psychiatric diagnoses via standardized instruments in order to develop a comprehensive model of impact for affected children and families. The value of the current report lies in the serial neuropsychological evaluations in individuals which demonstrate the clinical impact of ESES. Controlled trials in ESES are required to help determine what might be the most effective treatments. Recently, the RESCUE ESES international European collaboration has developed such a trial. Unfortunately, due to the rarity of the condition, the challenges of delivering multi-centre international trials (see Gentry et al., 2018), and variability in resources to support the trial assessments, this study has not recruited as well as planned. It is possible that international agreements between collaborating centres to collect data and manage patients in a limited number of standardized paradigms might be the most practical way to generate sufficient clinically useful data on treatment efficacy.

The implications of our study are that whilst some children experience stagnation in development, represented by a plateau in neuropsychological test scores and a corresponding decline in age-normative standard scores, others experience a more significant decline in cognitive functions consistent with an active disease process. In this group of children with ESES with a variety of underlying aetiologies and treatments, the underlying encephalopathy resulted in an insidious decline in cognitive ability. It is therefore important that children with ESES have early and continuing neuropsychological assessment and that developmental monitoring is linked with appropriate psychological, social and psychiatric support to improve mental wellbeing and social participation. Families and educational services should also be provided with accurate information to inform prognosis and support in relation to maximizing learning potential and social integration with peers.

Current treatment options for Encephalopathy related to Status Epilepticus during slow Sleep

Floor E. Jansen, Marina Nikanorova, Maria Peltola

Almost 50 years have elapsed since the first description of Encephalopathy related to Status Epilepticus during slow Sleep (ESES) (Patry et al., 1971), and a well-defined treatment protocol of this condition is still lacking. There is no general agreement whether immunomodulation, benzodiazepines or antiepileptic drugs (AEDs) should be used as a first-choice medication. Nor is there consensus on the duration of treatment after which improvement may be expected, and how long treatment needs to be continued after improvement is achieved. Treatment goals in ESES include seizure control, reduction of EEG abnormalities and most importantly potential improvement, or at least prevention, of further cognitive decline. The beneficial effect of treatment on both seizure frequency and severity and on cognitive functions in relation to the reduction of epileptiform discharges in sleep has been demonstrated in many studies (Aeby et al., 2005; Inutsuka et al., 2006; Kramer et al., 2009; Sanchez Fernandez et al., 2012).

The current treatment options for ESES include "routine" AEDs, benzodiazepines, immune modulation therapy, including corticosteroids, and surgical treatment.

■ Antiepileptic drugs

The most commonly used AEDs are sodium valproate, ethosuximide, sultiame and levetiracetam, though their effects are often temporary, partial or limited to control of clinical seizures. In a series by Inutsuka et al. (2006), 10 out of 15 patients (67%) responded with long-lasting seizure control and partial recovery of cognitive functions after treatment with valproate alone or in combination with ethosuximide. Liukkonen et al (2010) demonstrated efficacy of a combination of valproate and ethosuximide in two patients. Other investigators could not confirm these positive effects (Capovilla et al., 2004; Scholtes et al., 2005; Kramer et al., 2009).

Several studies have supported efficacy of levetiracetam in ESES treatment (Capovilla et al., 2004; Aeby et al., 2005; Wang et al., 2008; Atkins and Nikanorova, 2011; Larsson *et al.*, 2012). Capovilla *et al.* (2004) observed efficacy in two of three children (all with focal structural epilepsy and ESES), followed for 15 and 12 months, respectively. Aeby *et al.* (2005) reported EEG improvement in seven of 12 children after two months of treatment, and neuropsychological or behaviour improvement in nine. In their study, levetiracetam had been discontinued after one year in four patients because of ESES relapse while on treatment.

Wang *et al.* (2008) demonstrated levetiracetam efficacy in 5 of 6 children, but 2 of 5 responders relapsed after four and five months, respectively. In a study by Atkins and Nikanorova (2011), eight out of 20 patients demonstrated a long-lasting response (more than 12 months), and three showed a partial response (6-12 months). Nine had seizures prior to levetiracetam treatment initiation. Six became seizure-free when levetiracetam was added, and in three children a significant reduction of seizure frequency was observed. The authors emphasized the higher levetiracetam efficacy in patients with structural etiology compared to unknown and genetic etiology. Sultiame has been reported as effective in small series (Wirrell *et al.*, 2006; Kramer *et al.*, 2009).

Recently, one study reported a very significant effect of topiramate; 16 of 21 patients showed clinical and behavioural improvement at three months, with long lasting effect in 10 (Vrielynck *et al.*, 2017). Acetazolamide was reported to yield subjective clinical improvement in 5 of 6 children in whom up to 12 previous treatments had failed, when studied retrospectively (Fine *et al.*, 2015). Amantidine, although not considered to have anticonvulsive effects, became of interest because of the identified *GRIN2A* variant in patients with ESES which has recently been reported in a series of 20 patients with ESES. The SW index was found to have dropped from a mean of 76% to 53% and subjective cognitive, linguistic, or behavioral benefit was noted in the majority of patients (Wilson *et al.*, 2018).

Benzodiazepines demonstrate efficacy in the short term. Treatment with short cycles of high-dose diazepam (1-3 weeks) can lead to transient remission, but relapses necessitate repeated cycles (Inutsuka *et al.*, 2006; Kramer *et al.*, 2009). Kramer *et al.* (2009) reported a temporary response in three of eight patients after treatment with oral diazepam 0.75-1 mg/kg/day for three weeks, with a relapse within six months. In a series by Sanchez Fernandez *et al.* (2012), the mean spike wave index decreased from 77 to 41% in 29 patients with ESES after administration of 1 mg/kg oral diazepam every evening. In another study, valproate and benzodiazepines were not effective in nine out of 10 patients, and 3 patients experienced an adverse behavioural reaction (Scholtes *et al.*, 2005). Chronic treatment with oral clobazam in combination with other AEDs may have a sustained effect (Larrieu *et al.*, 1986). Recently, nine patients showed significant reduction of sleep spike waves after three months or daily clobazam 0.5 mg/kg (Vega *et al.*, 2018). Verbal IQ scores improved, although median IQ had not changed due to an unexplained decrease in non-verbal IQ in this series.

■ Ketogenic diet

The data on ketogenic diet in ESES treatment are limited. Bergqvist *et al.* (1997) described three patients with Landau-Kleffner syndrome refractory to traditional therapy. All three children showed improvement of their language performance, behaviour, and seizure frequency for 26, 24, and 12 months, respectively. In another study (Nikanorova *et al.*, 2009), the ketogenic diet did not appear to influence the neuropsychological outcome of ESES. Only one out of 5 patients responded with complete ESES resolution. More recently, two series were added to the literature. The combination of the KD with steroids was studied in 13 children (Ville et al., 2015). Of the patients, 61% were considered responders, but only one was able to discontinue steroids during follow-up. In a series by Reyes et al. (2015), 12 patients with ESES were treated with the ketogenic diet for a minimum of 18 months. At the end of follow-up, seven patients remained on the diet, one patient became seizure-free, and three had a significant improvement in seizure reduction. Efficacy of the ketogenic diet has been reviewed by Kelley and Kossoff in 2016. Of the 38 reported children, 41% had >50% seizure reduction, 45% had cognitive improvement, 53% had EEG improvement but only 9% had EEG normalization. Efficacy of the ketogenic diet in ESES may result from its anti-inflammatory potential or by increasing GABA that may be particularly important since GABAergic neurons in the thalamus may be damaged in patients with ESES (Kelley and Kossof, 2016).

■ Activation of the immune system in patients with ESES and response to immunomodulating treatment

A growing body of evidence has recently confirmed a link between epilepsy and inflammation. Various findings indicate the involvement of the immune system, including reduced serum levels of IgA and IgG subclasses but also elevated cerebrospinal fluid levels of IgG, IgM, as well as positive antinuclear antibodies, antibrain, antimyelin, and antiglutamate receptor antibodies in serum (Boscolo et al., 2005; Connolly et al., 2006; de Vries et al., 2016). The inflammatory process is mediated by cytokines, chemokines and proteases. To date, IL-1beta and HMGB1 overexpression has been found in resected focal cortical dysplasia, mesial temporal sclerosis and tubers (Connolly et al., 2006). Further, increased levels of IL-6 have been found in a number of epilepsy-related etiologies making it a consistent finding. However, there are only two studies of ESES that investigated cytokine profiles (Lehtimaki et al., 2011; van den Munckhof et al., 2016). Van den Munckhof found significantly higher levels of IL-1α, IL-6, IL-10, chemokine (C-C motif) ligand (CCL)2 and chemokine (C-X-C motif) ligand (CXCL)8/IL-8 in 11 patients with ESES as compared to controls. Further, IL-6 changes were accompanied by clear improvement of electroencephalography (EEG) patterns and neuropsychological evaluation after immunomodulating treatment. As seizures may be infrequent in ESES, it is suggested unlikely that IL-6 elevation and chronic inflammatory system activation result from recurrent seizures alone. Although it has been suggested that continuous epileptiform activity may also cause inflammatory system activation, the exact relationship- cause or consequence- is not known.

In addition to measuring the inflammatory process, effective response to immunomodulating therapy in patients with ESES provides further evidence for the role of immune system activation (Walker and Sills, 2012), although the mechanisms of action are not completely understood.

■ Intravenuous immunoglobins (IVIG)

IVIG was first used in the treatment of childhood epilepsy in 1977 (Pechadre et al., 1977). Since then, successful treatments with intravenous immunoglobulin (IVIG) in LKS or

CSWS/ESES syndrome have been published in a few case reports (Pechadre et al., 1977; Fayad et al., 1997; Mikati et al., 2002; Arts et al., 2009). Arts et al. reported the use of IVIG in six children with LKS or CSWS/ESES who were studied in a prospective manner. Only one of the six patients showed a clear, temporal, positive response to IVIG. The other children did not respond, and four of them were treated subsequently with prednisone.

■ Corticosteroids

Corticosteroids seem to offer better efficacy and more long-lasting effect than conventional AEDs. Different steroid modalities and schemes have been reported over years and again, results are mostly restricted to small case series. Lerman et al. described successful long-term treatment of ACTH and corticosteroids in four patients (Lerman et al., 1991). Repeated pulses with intravenous methylprednisolone was effective in two patients (Tsuru et al., 2000); they showed a maintenance of improved language performance with subsequent continuous oral prednisolone administration. Another nine out of ten patients manifested significant long-lasting improvement in language, cognition, and behavior after 6 months treatment with oral prednisolone 1 mg/kg/day (Sinclair and Snyder, 2005). Only few and reversible side effects were noted. Haberlandt et al. (2010) showed that pulsatile corticoid therapy with dexamethasone was an effective alternative treatment to adrenocorticotropic hormone for a number of epilepsy syndromes, including ESES. Dexamethasone was also considered effective in a study by Chen et al. (2016) with seven out of 15 responders, although relapses were seen in 4 when dexamethasone was discontinued after one month. Kramer et al (2009) concluded that the 64% (11 of 17 patients) short-term efficacy of steroid therapy was greater than the efficacy of any other agents (including AEDs, benzodiazepines and immunoglobulins). However, of those, 33% eventually relapsed and 22% became steroid dependent. Two centers combined their experience with corticosteroid treatment in a large retrospective cohort of 44 patients with CSWS or LKS (Buzato et al., 2009). All but two patients were administered daily hydrocortisone, in a scheme lasting up to 21 months. Initial positive response was found in 34 of 44 patients (77.2%), with normalization of the EEG in 21 patients. Although relapses occurred (14 of 34), 20 patients (45.4%) were found to be long-term responders. Higher IQ/DQ and shorter CSWS duration were significantly related to positive treatment response. Recently, the electroclinical spectrum and treatment efficacy was reported in a large cohort of 44 Turkish patients with ESES (Gencpinar et al., 2016). Patients treated with a minimum of two AEDs did not differ from patients treated with AEDs and ACTH with respect to seizure outcome, SWI and cognitive outcome. On the other hand, van den Munckhof et al. (2018) and Altunel et al. (2017) did find steroid treatment to be most successful. Altunel reported the effects on SWI in sleep EEGs and ADHD symptoms in 75 patients treated with ACTH (with repeated cycles when SWI remained > 15%). They found a reduction in SWI in all the patients that was accompanied by a mean improvement of 67% in ADHD-like symptoms after treatment with ACTH. Van den Munckhof reported improved cognitive performance in a series of 47 patients with ESES. More so, improvement of daily functioning after treatment was strongly associated with SWI decrease. Pooling individual patient data yielded treatment success (for EEG or cognitive improvement) in 81% of ESES cases for steroids, as compared to 68% for benzodiazepines and 49% for other AEDs (van den Munckhof et al., 2015).

Epilepsy surgery

Hemispherectomy and lobar or multilobar resection has been found effective for selected children and adolescents with a congenital or early-acquired brain lesion, despite abundant generalized or bilateral epileptiform discharges on EEG (Wyllie et al., 2007). Pooled data from several studies shows the effect of 14 hemispherectomies or hemispherotomies and four resections in patients with structural and pharmacoresistant ESES (Wyllie et al., 2007; Battaglia et al., 2009; Kallay et al., 2009; Loddenkemper et al., 2009; Roulet-Perez et al., 2010; Peltola et al., 2011; Fournier-Del Castillo et al., 2014). Fifteen of 18 patients had strictly unilateral brain lesions. In the other patients, the lesion was predominantly unilateral. The etiology of lesions was perinatal vascular with or without thalamic injury in the majority of the patients. Two of 18 patients presented with hemispheric or lobar polymicrogyria. Age at the hemispherotomy or hemispherectomy varied between 3.6 and 6.2 years (median: 6.9 years), and at the resection between 4.7-14.9 years (median: 4.9 years). Minimum duration of postsurgical follow-up was 18 months. Good response after surgery was seen with seizure freedom in 14 of 17 patients with preoperative seizures, resolution of ESES in all except one patient, who had residual regional ESES, and behavioural and cognitive improvement in all. Cognitive catch-up with increment of IQ or DQ with greater than or equal to 10 points was verified by comparable pre- and postoperative IQ/DQ measurements in nine of 14 patients after hemispherotomy or hemispherectomy and in three of four patients after resection. In 2017, Jeong et al. (2017) reported hemispherotomy resulting in complete seizure control in all nine children with ESES and resolution of continuous spike-and-wave discharge in six of six patients in whom postoperative EEG recordings were available. Regression of skills was stopped in all patients and in four of them developmental and academic gains were noted in parental reports.

Factors that are suggestive of favorable outcome are a strictly unilateral MRI lesion in patients considered for resective or disconnective surgery, preoperative propagation of SES from one hemisphere to another and normal or near-normal cognitive development before or at the diagnosis of ESES (Loddenkemper et al., 2009; Roulet-Perez et al., 2010; Peltola et al., 2011). The meta-analysis by van den Munckhof confirms surgery to be the most effective treatment in patients with structural etiology (van den Munckhof et al, 2015).

Conclusions

In patients with ESES, different treatment regimens have been advised and responses are unpredictable. Here, we reviewed the current literature. Many of the studies are small or retrospective, and may have been published only because of an exceptionally good or bad treatment effect. Next, most of these studies used qualitative outcome data only, not analyzing structured and serial neuropsychological assessments. Furthermore, series published to date used very different schemes of steroid treatment, making comparisons difficult. Finally, data on relapse rates and adverse events were largely missing.

Based on the comprehensive review of the literature and our own clinical experience, we propose a therapeutic approach (*figure 1*). Since epilepsy surgery was found to be most effective, children with ESES due to unilateral structural abnormalities should be discussed for surgery immediately. We propose to start with clobazam in patients without regression but

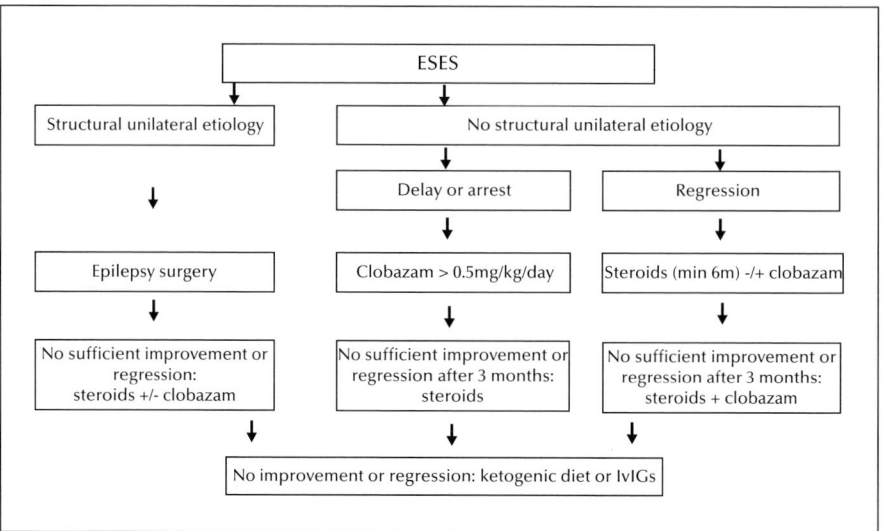

Figure 1/ Flow chart of therapeutic approach, based on review of the literature and expert opinion.

consider steroids in cases who regressed. In addition to this flow chart, individual choices can be made depending on the epilepsy syndrome, for example sultiam could be first chosen in children with atypical benign focal epilepsy of childhood and ethosuximide could be effective in children with solitary thalamic injury. Further research to provide definite answers regarding treatment of children with ESES is warranted. For this goal, a European randomized controlled trial has been undertaken. RESCUE ESES (Randomized European trial of Steroids *versus* Clobazam Usage for Encephalopathy related to Status Epilepticus during slow Sleep) is a multicenter trial comparing treatment with either corticosteroids or clobazam in newly diagnosed patients. Quantitative cognitive and EEG outcome and possible predictors of treatment response will be assessed.

Encephalopathy related to Status Epilepticus during slow Sleep: current concepts and future directions

Carlo Alberto Tassinari, Guido Rubboli

Encephalopathy related to Status Epilepticus during slow Sleep (ESES), otherwise labelled as "continuous spike and waves during sleep (CSWS)" was first reported more than 45 years ago. Since then, a considerable wealth of clinical observations and neurophysiological, neuroimaging, and genetic findings have been accumulated. However, in spite of this abundance of information, several issues related to ESES, not least the very definition of this condition, are still debated. In this paper, we discuss, in the light of current knowledge and some recent research, some aspects relevant to the delineation and identification of this condition to further understand pathophysiological mechanisms; we will also outline possible lines for future research.

■ The definition of ESES

There is a large consensus that the cardinal feature of ESES, *i.e.* Encephalopathy related to Status Epilepticus during slow Sleep, is the appearance of, or worsening of previously present cognitive disorders and behavioural disturbances in association with the occurrence of a striking activation of EEG epileptic abnormalities during REM sleep (see also Hirsch *et al.*, p.7-16, and Tassinari and Rubboli, p.17-18). This central concept for the diagnosis of ESES, that has been proposed since 1977 (Tassinari *et al.*, 1977) and that is incorporated in the 2010 ILAE definition of epileptic encephalopathy (Berg *et al.*, 2010), needs to be reaffirmed. Indeed, as shown by a recent survey (Sanchez Fernandez *et al.*, 2013), about 60% of American pediatric neurologists and epileptologists consider the demonstration of cognitive and/or language regression not mandatory, and a further 6-13% not relevant, for the diagnosis of ESES/CSWS. We believe that ESES can be diagnosed only when there is evidence of a deterioration of the cognitive and behavioural status in concomitance with the occurrence of extremely abundant epileptic discharges during NREM sleep. In our opinion, the observation of an exaggeration of epileptic activity during NREM sleep, without any demonstration of a clinical effect, *i.e.* appearance or worsening of an encephalopathy, does not allow the diagnosis of ESES. This clinical-EEG correlation can be a complex task due to:

- a) the heterogeneity of neuropsychological disorders, such as attention deficit, decreased IQ, language disorders, disturbances in spatial and temporal orientation, and memory impairment, as well as motor disorders (see review by Tassinari *et al.*, 2019);
- b) a preexisting cognitive and behavioural derangement, that in most severe cases, can render a clinical/neuropsychological assessment challenging even before the appearance of ESES;
- c) an extremely selective cognitive impairment which can occur in cases with very focal ESES (Kuki *et al.*, 2014).

These difficulties demand the development of appropriate neuropsychological testing, individually tailored to specific deficits and possibly complemented by adequate neurophysiological and neuroimaging data (Filippini *et al.*, 2013; Tassinari *et al.*, 2015).

The proteiform clinical features of the encephalopathies have been extensively described (Panayiotopoulos, 1999; Galanoupoulos *et al.*, 2000; Hughes 2010). Three main groups can be retained:

- a) a " pervasive" group with patients with concomitant impairment of language, memory, spatial orientation and with ADHD and autistic-like behaviors;
- b) a "combined" group with patients with multiple concomitant dysfunctions, with one domain most clinically impaired, *e.g.* language as in LKS, or mainly a "frontal", "occipital", or "parietal" dysfunction, with spatio-temporal or motor disturbances such as negative myoclonus, dyspraxias, and gait disorders (Billard *et al.*, 1982; Roulet Peretz 1993; Neville *et al.*, 1998);
- c) a selective group with patients with a unique (as documented so far) specific impairment, as " a visual agnosia", as reported by Eriksson *et al.* (2003), or " a selective dysgraphia" as reported by Kuki *et al.* (2014). The dysfunction of a very restricted patch of cortex, or even of a limited number of cortical columns, could thus result in such a selective impairment which could be easily overlooked, challenging a precise and correct clinical assessment (Tassinari *et al.*, 2015).

Obviously, the "pervasive", "combined" and "selective" groups are static "frames" of an evolutive multifactorial age-related condition. The same patient could possibly evolve from an initial selective impairment to a combined or pervasive condition and eventually reverse, not necessarily in that order, to a previous stage, when partial remissions and relapses occur during the evolution.

During ESES, epileptic seizures are reported in the majority of cases, however, it is accepted that some cases have no history of clinical seizures at all. Therefore, the presence of epilepsy cannot be considered a mandatory feature for the diagnosis of ESES.

Atypical evolution from benign childhood epilepsy with centro-temporal spikes (BCECTS) to ESES or LKS has been reported (Saltik *et al.*, 2005; Kramer *et al.*, 2009; Tovia *et al.*, 2011; see also Caraballo *et al.*, p. 19-24). Some studies that have identified possible prognostic factors predicting an atypical evolution from BCECTS to ESES or LKS (Fejerman et al., 2000; Massa et al., 2001; Saltik et al., 2005) need to be confirmed by further data in larger populations. Actually, BCECTS and ESES have been suggested to represent the more benign and the more severe end of a spectrum encompassing childhood focal epilepies respectively, in which the positioning along this spectrum might be influenced by a complex interplay between brain development, maturation processes and susceptibility genes (Rudolf et al., 2009; Carvill, 2013; Lemke et al., 2013; Lesca et al., 2013; Lesca et al., p. 49-53). These concepts introduce the role of genetic factors in the etiology of ESES. However, this latter point further emphasizes the need for a shared and accepted definition of ESES and of its diagnostic criteria that allows precise genotype-phenotype associations.

ESES, or CSWS, or....?

In its original description, Tassinari's group referred to the condition now labelled as ESES/CSWS as "Subclinical electrical status epilepticus induced by sleep in children" (Patry et al., 1971). At that time, the strict link between the peculiar EEG pattern during sleep and the cognitive/behavioural disturbances was not immediately appreciated, therefore the term "subclinical" was used. The concept that this sleep-related exaggerated epileptic activity was not "subclinical" but was indeed "clinical", producing an encephalopathy, was proposed in 1977, when Tassinari et al. (1977) reported 11 additional patients and the term "encephalopathy related to status epilepticus during slow sleep" (*i.e.* ESES) was coined (see also Tassinari and Rubboli, p. 17-18). Later on, the term "Epilepsy with continuous spikes and waves during slow sleep (ECSWS)" was introduced to refer to the same group of patients (Tassinari et al., 1985; Panayiotopoulos, 2005). The International League Against Epilepsy (ILAE) adopted the term "Continuous spikes and waves during sleep (CSWS)", and accepted that a similar EEG pattern could be associated also with Landau-Kleffner syndrome (Commission on Classification and Terminology of the International League Against Epilepsy, 1989; Engel, 2006). More recently, the term "Epileptic encephalopathy with continuous spike and waves during sleep" has been used by the Commission on Classification and Terminology of the ILAE (Engel, 2006; Berg et al., 2010). Even though these different terms were not accompanied by any defining criteria of the syndrome, we can assume that these diverse and partially overlapping terms have been used to define the same or very similar conditions.

The assessment of the EEG during sleep

Since the first description by Patry et al. (1971), a spike-wave index (SWI) during NREM sleep, defined as the percentage of time occupied by spike and wave discharges, was used to provide an objective measure of the amount of epileptic activity during sleep. In the six patients reported originally by Tassinari's group (Patry et al., 1971), the lowest SWI was 85% and since then this value has been considered the threshold over which a diagnosis of ESES could be made. Over the years, many different studies have used considerably different SWI, whose threshold could vary from 25% to 90% (reviewed by Scheltens-de Boer, 2009; see also Cantalupo et al., p. 37-48, and Gardella et al., p. 25-36). However, rarely these studies report a clear description of the methods to measure the SWI, or which type (in terms of morphology and topography) of sleep-related epileptic discharges were assessed. Furthermore, recording setting (overnight EEG *versus* daytime sleep EEG) and length of the recording varies considerably in the different investigations.

Several pieces of evidence have shown that, in subjects in whom a striking activation of epileptic abnormalities occurs during sleep in comparison to wakefulness, a cognitive/behavioural derangement can occur with SWI lower than 85%. Therefore, the concept of a minimum SWI necessary for the diagnosis of ESES can be flexible, and not rigidly delimited by a SWI threshold >85%, once the main feature of ESES, *i.e.* occurrence of cognitive deterioration associated with sleep-enhanced epileptic activity, is demonstrated. This implies that the diagnosis of ESES cannot depend solely on the assessment of the SWI but it requires a precise correlation with the clinical picture. These concepts in some respect apply also to the spike topography, in particular in focal ESES, once there is evidence that a more or less selective neuropsychological deficit can be related to an enhanced focal-multifocal epileptic EEG activity during sleep in the cortical area involved in the performance of that neuropsychological task (Kuki *et al.*, 2014; Tassinari *et al.*, 2015). This conforms to the concept underlying the definition of ESES, *i.e.* disruption of cognitive functions in relation to increased epileptic activity during sleep in the cortical areas involved in the disrupted cognitive processes.

■ Is ESES a model of cognitive deterioration caused by impaired NREM sleep homeostasis?

Following the concepts just mentioned above, the evidence that in ESES a cognitive/behavioural derangement can be observed with very different SWIs, and sometimes without a linear correlation between the severity of the encephalopathic picture and the SWI value, suggest that other parameters besides SWI might be relevant to further understand the relationships between the peculiar sleep EEG pattern and the clinical, *i.e.* encephalopathic, picture. Recent data suggest that the negative effects of ESES may depend on the impairment of synaptic homeostasis processes occurring during normal sleep which are particularly important in the developmental age. The synaptic homeostasis hypothesis (SHY) proposes that synaptic strength increases within neuronal networks during wakefulness (*e.g.* due to learning processes) and is renormalized or downscaled during sleep through synaptic weakening/elimination (Tononi and Cirelli, 2014). Changes in synaptic strength are reflected in the EEG by changes of sleep slow wave activity. In ESES, an impairment of synaptic downscaling has been demonstrated by Bolsterli and Huber (2011, 2014) (see also Rubboli *et al.*, p. 69-76). In addition, they have shown that an altered overnight decrease of slow wave slope - a sign of altered slow wave homeostasis -during ESES improves with remission of ESES (Bolsterli *et al.*, 2017). Indeed, this study suggests that the SWI may not be the only parameter that should be investigated in ESES, and a derangement of homeostatic sleep processes, as measured by the decline of the slope of sleep slow waves, might better reflect the severity of the cognitive derangement. These findings suggest a fascinating as well as likely pathogenic mechanism: the prolonged paroxysmal activity (during around eight hours of sleep per day for several months up to a number of years) could interfere with the changes in sleep slow wave activity that normally occur in the course of sleep and this may be causally related to impairment in cognitive functions and behavior associated with ESES (Tassinari and Rubboli, 2006; Rubboli *et al.*, p. 69-76).

Other physiological graphoelements of sleep have been recently shown to play a role in the consolidation of memory and maintenance of cognitive function. In particular, sleep spindle activity has been demonstrated to be associated with different aspects of cognitive performance in children, and variation in spindle activity in adult sleep may shed light on the role of this sleep signature in the developmental age (Chatburn *et al.*, 2013; Reynolds *et al.*, 2018; Vermeulen *et al.*, 2018). In ESES, lack or decrement of physiological sleep features, such as spindles, might be an additional factor impairing the remodelling of neuronal networks subserving cognitive processes, that normally occur during sleep.

This evidence introduces new methodological perspectives for the analysis of the electro-clinical correlations in ESES and opens new avenues to investigate and further understand this syndrome, providing a novel approach to elucidate the relevance of sleep-related paroxysmal activities, not only for ESES, but for a large population of children with significant activation of epileptic activity during sleep.

■ Critical periods and plasticity as relevant age-related variables in the pathophysiology of ESES

As thoughtfully discussed by Issa (2014), the model of critical periods (as proposed by Hubel and Wiesel, 1970) can further contribute to the understanding of the neurobiology of ESES. According to Issa (2014):

- *"there are in childhood critical-sensitive periods allowing the cortex to adapt to the idiosyncrasies of individuals and their environment;... Although the exact age range that covers the language critical periods... is often debated,... the age at which Landau-Kleffner patients have electrographic seizures falls within the commonly agreed critical periods [...];*

- *"In ESES, the organisation of cortex is driven into an abnormal structure by state-dependent (sleep) epileptiform activity during the critical period, but the abnormal electrical activity stops, once the critical period is over [...].*

Since the cognitive and behavioral disorders start and end at nearly the same time as the start and end of the critical periods, these disturbances appear to be strongly linked to these periods, that are crucial for normal development. According to Issa's hypothesis, the "electrical status epilepticus" would drive maladaptive plasticity during these critical periods; the termination of these periods would cement those adaptive changes, thus explaining the long-lasting effects of ESES on cortical functions (Issa, 2014). In addition, during these periods, the role of NREM sleep is extremely relevant for brain plasticity, and this can explain why sleep disruption does not just prevent new acquisitions but would actually degrade previously developed cortical structures (Frank *et al.*, 2001). In ESES, this could hinder the physiological switch from one hemisphere to another or it could result in a redistribution of functions across different cortical areas at an early age (Issa, 2014).

The complexity and variability that characterize the ESES syndrome, as we have underlined above, render the diagnosis hazardous based on a single semiological component. The amount of paroxysmal activity during sleep, "the spike and wave index", within the appropriate clinical context could be misleading. Further parameters are needed in order to elucidate the natural history of ESES. The contribution of new neuroimaging techniques, such as diffusion tensor imaging tractography, to explore age-dependent differences and heritability of the perisylvian language network (Budisavlievic *et al.*, 2015), altered white matter connectivity (Ameis and Catani, 2015; Catani *et al.*, 2016) or networks related to behavior, cognitive and motor tasks (Catani *et al.*, 2013; Parlatini *et al.*, 2017) might add new perspectives in the study of ESES. Moving from hodology to function (Catani, 2007) could be a rewarding route towards further understanding of this fascinating condition.

References

Abreu R, Leite M, Leal A, Figueiredo P. Objective selection of epilepsy-related independent components from EEG data. *J Neurosci Methods* 2015;258:67–78.

Acherman P. EEG analysis applied to sleep. *Epileptologie* 2009;26:28–33.

Aeby A, Poznanski N, Verheulpen D, et al. Levetiracetam efficacy in epileptic syndromes with continuous spikes and waves during slow sleep: experience in 12 cases. *Epilepsia* 2015;46:1937–42.

Agarwal R, Kumar A, Tiwari VN, Chugani H. Thalamic abnormalities in children with continuous spike-wave during slow-wave sleep: An F-18-fluorodeoxyglucose positron emission tomography perspective. *Epilepsia* 2016;57:263–71.

Allen AS, Berkovic SF, Cossette P, et al. De novo mutations in epileptic encephalopathies. *Nature* 2013;501(7466):217–21.

Altunel A, Altunel EÖA, Sever A. Response to adrenocorticotropic in attention deficit hyperactivity disorder-like symptoms in electrical status epilepticus in sleep syndrome is related to electroencephalographic improvement: A retrospective study. *Epilepsy Behav* 2017;74:161–6.

Ameis SH, Catani M. Altered white matter connectivity as a neural substrate for social impairment in Autism Spectrum Disorder. *Cortex* 2015;62:158–81.

Amzica F, Steriade M. Electrophysiological correlates of sleep delta waves. *Electroencephalogr Clin Neurophysiol* 1998;107:69–83.

Amzica F, Steriade M. Neuronal and glial membrane potentials during sleep and paroxysmal oscillations in the neocortex. *J Neurosci* 2000;20:6648–65.

Amzica F. Physiology of sleep and wakefulness as it relates to the physiology of epilepsy. *J Clin Neurophysiol* 2002;19:488–503.

Arts WF, Aarsen FK, Scheltens-de Boer M, Catsman-Berrevoets CE. Landau-Kleffner syndrome and CSWS syndrome: treatment with intravenous immunoglobulins. *Epilepsia* 2009;5(7):55–8.

Arzimanoglou A, Cross H. Cognitive impairment and behavioral disorders in Encephalopathy related to Status Epilepticus during slow Sleep : diagnostic assessment and outcome. In: Encephalopathy related to Status Epilepticus during slow Sleep: linking epilepsy, sleep disruption and cognitive impairment. Rubboli G, Tassinari CA, editors. Montrouge: John Libbey Eurotext; 2020. p. 77–81.

Atkins M, Nikanorova M. A prospective study of levetiracetam efficacy in epileptic syndromes with continuous spike-waves during slow sleep. *Seizure* 2011;20:635–9.

Azcona G, Gurtubay IG, Mosquera A, et al. Estudio comparativo entre tres sistemas de cuantificación del índice de punta-onda en pacientes con punta-onda continua del sueño lento. *Rev Neurol* 2017;65:439–46.

Ballaban-gil K, Goldberg R, Moshe SL, Shinnar S. EEG evaluation and treatment of children with language regression. *Epilepsia* 1998;39:156.

Battaglia D, Veggiotti P, Lettori D, et al. Functional hemispherectomy in children with epilepsy and CSWS due to unilateral early brain injury including thalamus: sudden recovery of CSWS. *Epilepsy Res* 2009;87:290–8.

Beaumanoir A, Ballis T, Varfis G, Ansari K. Benign epilepsy of childhood with rolandic spikes. A clinical, electroencephalographic, and telencephalographic study. *Epilepsia* 1974;15:301–15.

Beaumanoir A, Bureau M, Deonna T, Mira L, Tassinari CA. *Continuous spikes and waves during slow sleep. Electrical status epilepticus during slow sleep.* London: John Libbey; 1995.

Beaumanoir A. EEG Data. In: *Continuous spikes and waves during slow sleep.* Beaumanoir A, Bureau T, Deonna T, Mira L, Tassinari CA. Oxford: John Libbey & Company Ltd; 1995. p. 217–23.

Beelke M, Nobili L, Baglietto MG, et al. Relationship of sigma activity to sleep interictal epileptic discharges: a study in children affected by benign epilepsy with occipital paroxysms. *Epilepsy Res* 2000;40:179–86.

Beenhakker MP, Huguenard JR. Neurons that fire together also conspire together: is normal sleep circuitry hijacked to generate epilepsy? *Neuron* 2009;62:612–32.

Beniczky S, Hirsch LJ, Kaplan PW, et al. Unified EEG terminology and criteria for nonconvulsive status epilepticus. *Epilepsia* 2013;54(6):28–9.

Ben-Zeev B, Kivity S, Pshitizki Y, Watemberg N, Brand N, Kramer U. Congenital hydrocephalus and continuous spike wave in slow-wave sleep a common association? *J Child Neurol* 2004;19:129–34.

Berg AT, Berkovic SF, Brodie MJ, et al. Revised terminology and concepts for organization of seizures and epilepsies: report of the ILAE Commission on Classification and Terminology, 2005-2009. *Epilepsia* 2010;51:676–85.

Bergqvist AGC, Brooks-Kayal AR. Ketogenic diet in the treatment of acquired epileptic aphasia. *Ann Neurol* 1997;42:504.

Berkovic SF, Mulley JC, Scheffer IE, Petrou S. Human epilepsies: interaction of genetic and acquired factors. *Trends Neurosci* 2006;29(7):391–7.

Billard C, Autret A, Laffont F, Lucas B, Degiovanni E. Electrical status epilepticus during sleep in children: a reappraisal from eight new cases. In: *Sleep and epilepsy.* Sterman MB, Shouse MN, Passouant P. London and New York: Academic Press; 1982. p. 481–91.

Binnie CD. Significance and management of transitory cognitive impairment due to subclinical EEG discharges in children. *Brain & Dev* 1993;15(1):23–30.

Blume WT, Pillay N. Electrographic and clinical correlates of secondary bilateral synchrony. *Epilepsia* 1985;26:636–41.

Bobbili DR, Lal D, May P, et al. Exome-wide analysis of mutational burden in patients with typical and atypical Rolandic epilepsy. *Eur J Hum Genet* 2018;26(2):258–64.

Boelsterli BK, Gardella E, Pavlidis E, et al. Remission of encephalopathy with status epilepticus (ESES) during sleep renormalizes regulation of slow wave sleep. *Epilepsia* 2017;58:1892–901.

Bölsterli BK, Fattinger S, Kurth S, et al. Spike wave location and density disturb sleep slow waves in patients with CSWS (continuous spike waves during sleep). *Epilepsia* 2014;55(4):584–91.

Bolsterli BK, Schmitt B, Bast T, et al. Impaired slow wave sleep downscaling in encephalopathy with status epilepticus during sleep (ESES). *Clin Neurophysiol* 2011;122:1779–87.

Boly M, Jones B, Findlay G, et al. Altered sleep homeostasis correlates with cognitive impairment in patients with focal epilepsy. *Brain* 2017;140:1026–40.

Borbely AA, Achermann P. Sleep homeostasis and models of sleep regulation. In: *Principles and practice of sleep medicine*. Kryger MH, Toth T, Dement WC. 4th Ed. Philadelphia: Elsevier Saunders; 2005. p. 405–17.

Boscolo S, Baldas V, Gobbi G, et al. Anti-brain but not celiac disease antibodies in Landau-Kleffner syndrome and related epilepsies. *J Neuroimmunol* 2005;160:228–32.

Brown R, Basheer R, Mckenna J, Strecker R, McCarley R. Control of sleep and wakefulness. *Physiol Rev* 2012;92:1087–187.

Broyd SJ, Demanuele C, Debener S, Helps SK, James CJ, Sonuga-Barke EJS. Default-mode brin dysfunction in mental disorders: A systematic review. *Neurosci Biobehav Rev* 2009;33:279–96.

Bruni O, Novelli L, Luchetti A, et al. Reduced NREM sleep instability in benign childhood epilepsy with centrotemporal spikes. *Clin Neurophysiol* 2010;121:665–71.

Buchmann A, Ringli M, Kurth S, et al. Sleep slow-wave activity as a mirror of cortical maturation. *Cereb Cortex* 2011;21:607–15.

Budisavlievic S, Dell'Acqua F, Rijsdijk VF, et al. Age related differences and Heritability of the Perisylvian Language Networks. *J Neurosci* 2015;35(37):12625–34.

Bureau M. Continuous spikes and waves during slow sleep (CSWS): definition of the syndrome. In: *Continuous spikes and waves during slow sleep: acquired epileptic aphasia and related conditions*. Beaumanoir A, Bureau M, Deonna T, et al. London: John Libbey; 1995. p. 17–26.

Bureau M. Outstanding cases of CSWS and LKS: analysis of the data sheets provided by the participants. In: *Continuous spike and waves during slow sleep. Electrical status epilepticus during slow sleep*. Beaumanoir A, Bureau M, Deonna T, Mira L, Tassinari CA. London: John Libby; 1995. p. 213–6.

Burnashev N, Szepetowski P. NMDA receptor subunit mutations in neurodevelopmental disorders. *Curr Opin Pharmacol* 2015;20:73–82.

Bushey D, Tononi G, Cirelli C. Sleep and synaptic homeostasis: structural evidence in Drosophila. *Science* 2011;332:1576–81.

Buzato M, Bulteau C, Altuzarra C, Dulac O, Van Bogaert P. Corticosteroids as treatment of epileptic syndromes with continuous spike-waves during slow-wave sleep. *Epilepsia* 2009;50(7):68–72.

Buzsaki G. Memory consolidation during sleep: a neurophysiological perspective. *J Sleep Res* 1998; 7(1):17–23.

Buzsaki G. Two-stage model of memory trace formation: a role for "noisy" brain states. *Neuroscience* 1989;31:551–70.

Campana C, Zubler F, Gibbs S, et al. Suppression of interictal spikes during phasic rapid eye movement sleep: a quantitative stereo-electroencephalography study. *J Sleep Res* 2017;26:606–13.

Campbell IG, Darchia N, Higgins LM, et al. Adolescent changes in homeostatic regulation of EEG activity in the delta and theta frequency bands during NREM sleep. *Sleep* 2011;34:83–91.

Campbell IG, Feinberg I. Longitudinal trajectories of nonrapid eye movement delta and theta EEG as indicators of adolescent brain maturation. *PNAS* 2009;106:5177–80.

Cantalupo G, Pavlidis E, Beniczky S, Gardella E, Larsson P. Quantitative EEG analysis in Encephalopathy related to Status Epilepticus during slow Sleep. In: Encephalopathy related to Status Epilepticus during slow Sleep: linking epilepsy, sleep disruption and cognitive impairment. Rubboli G, Tassinari CA, editors. Montrouge: John Libbey Eurotext; 2020. p. 37–48.

Cantalupo G, Rubboli G, Tassinari CA. In search of the Rosetta Stone for ESE.S. *Epilepsia* 2013;54:766–7.

Cantalupo G, Rubboli G, Tassinari CA. Night-time unravelling of the brain web: Impaired synaptic downscaling in ESES - The Penelope syndrome. *Clin Neurophysiol* 2011;122:1691–2.

Capovilla G, Beccaria F, Cagdas S, Montagnini A, Segala R, Paganelli D. Efficacy of levetiracetam in pharmacoresistant continuous spikes and waves during slow sleep. *Acta Neurol Scand* 2004;110: 144–7.

Caraballo R, Cejas N, Chamorro N, Kaltenmeier MC, Fortini S, Soprano AM. Landau-Kleffner syndrome: a study of 29 patients. *Seizures* 2014;23(2):98–104.

Caraballo R, Cersosimo R, Fejerman N. A particular type of epilepsy in children with congenital hemiparesis associated with unilateral polymicrogyria. *Epilepsia* 1999;40:865–71.

Caraballo R, Veggiotti P, Kaltenmeier MC, et al. Encephalopathy with status epilepticus during sleep or continuous spikes and waves during slow sleep syndrome: a multicenter, long-term follow-up study of 117 patients. *Epilepsy Res* 2013;105:164–73.

Caraballo RH, Aldao Mdel R, Cachia P. Benign childhood seizure susceptibility syndrome: three case reports. *Epileptic Disord* 2011;13(2):133–9.

Caraballo RH, Astorino F, Cersosimo R, Soprano AM, Fejerman N. Atypical evolution in childhood epilepsy with occipital paroxysms (Panayiotopoulos type). *Epileptic Disord* 2001;3:157–62.

Caraballo RH, Bongiorni L, Cersosimo R, Semprino M, Espeche A, Fejerman N. Epileptic encephalopathy with continuous spikes and waves during sleep in children with shunted hydrocephalus: a study of nine cases. *Epilepsia* 2008;49:1520–7.

Caraballo RH, Cersósimo RO, Fortini PS, et al. Congenital hemiparesis, unilateral polymicrogyria and epilepsy with or without status epilepticus during sleep: a study of 66 patients with long-term follow-up. *Epileptic Disord* 2013;15(4):417–27.

Caraballo RH, Fortini S, Flesler S, Pasteris MC, Caramuta L, Portuondo E. Encephalopathy with status epilepticus during sleep: unusual EEG patterns. *Seizure* 2015;25:117–25.

Carvill GL, Regan BM, Yendle SC, et al. GRIN2A mutations cause epilepsy-aphasia spectrum disorders. *Nat Genet* 2013;45(9):1073–6.

Catani M, Dell'Acqua F, Budisavljevic S, et al. Frontal networks in adults with autism spectrum disorder. *Brain* 2016;139:616–30.

Catani M, Mesulam MM, Jakobsen E, et al. A novel frontal pathway underlies verbal fluency in primary progressive aphasia. *Brain* 2013;136:2619–28.

Catani M. From hodology to function. *Brain* 2007;130:602–5.

Chan S, Baldeweg T, Cross JH. A role for sleep disruption in cognitive impairment in children with epilepsy. *Epilepsy Behav* 2011;2:435–40.

Chatburn A, Coussens S, Lushington K, Kennedy D, Baumert M, Kohler M. Sleep spindle activity and cognitive performance in healthy children. *Sleep* 2013;36:237–43.

Chavakula V, Sánchez Fernández I, Peters JM, et al. Automated quantification of spikes. *Epilepsy Behav* 2013;26(2):143–52.

Chen J, Cai F, Jiang L, Hu Y, Feng C. A prospective study of dexamethasone therapy in refractory epileptic encephalopathy with continuous spike-and-wave during sleep. *Epilepsy Behav* 2016;55:1–5.

Clemens B, Majoros E. Sleep studies in benign epilepsy of childhood with rolandic spikes. II. Analysis of discharge frequency and its relation to sleep dynamics. *Epilepsia* 1987;28:24–7.

Cloarec R, Bruneau N, Rudolf G, et al. PRRT2 links infantile convulsions and paroxysmal dyskinesia with migraine. *Neurology* 2012;79(21):2097–103.

Commission on Classification Terminology of the International League Against Epilepsy. Proposal for revised classification of epilepsies and epileptic syndromes. *Epilepsia* 1989;30:389–99.

Connolly AM, Chez M, Streif EM, et al. Brain-derived neurotrophic factor and autoantibodies to neural antigens in sera of children with autistic spectrum disorders, Landau-Kleffner syndrome, and epilepsy. *Biol Psychiatry* 2006;59:354–63.

Connolly AM, Chez MG, Pestronk A, Arnold ST, Mehta S, Deuel RK. Serum autoantibodies to brain in Landau-Kleffner variant, autism, and other neurologic disorders. *J Pediatr* 1999;134(5):607–13.

Cortinovis P, Badinand N, Bastuji H, Kocher L, Revol M. CSWS: SW index value according to the slow sleep stages. In: Continuous spikes and waves during slow sleep, electrical status epilepticus during slow sleep: acquired epileptic aphasia and related conditions. Beaumanoir M, Bureau M, Deonna T, Mira L, Tassinari CA. London, England: John Libbey & Co; 1995. p. 149–51.

Csercsa R, Dombovari B, Fabo D, et al. Laminar analysis of slow wave activity in humans. *Brain* 2010;133:2814–29.

Dalla Bernardina B, Bondavalli S, Colamaria V. Benign epilepsy of childhood with rolandic spikes (BERS) during sleep. In: *Sleep and Epilepsy*. Sterman MB, Shouse MN, Passouant P. New York: Academic Press; 1982. p. 495–506.

Dalla Bernardina B, Colamaria V, Capovilla P, Bondavalli S. Sleep and benign partial epilepsies of childhood. In: *Epilepsy, sleep and sleep deprivation*. Degen R, Niedermeyer E. Elsevier Science Publ: BV; 1984. p. 119–33.

Dalla Bernardina B, Fontana E, Michelizza B, Colamaria V, Capovilla G, Tassinari CA. Partial epilepsies of childhood, bilateral synchronization, continuous spike-waves during slow sleep. In: Manelis S, Bental E, Loeber JN, Dreifuss FE, eds. *Advances in epileptology. XVIIth epilepsy international symposium*. New York: Raven Press; 1989. p. 295–302.

Dalla Bernardina B, Sgro' V, Fejerman N. Epilepsy with centro-temporal spikes and related syndromes. In: *Epileptic syndromes in infancy, childhood and adolescence (4th Ed)*. Roger J, Bureau M, Dravet C, Genton P, Tassinari CA, Wolf P, editors. John Libbey Eurotext; 2005. p. 203–26.

Dalla Bernardina B, Tassinari CA, Dravet C, et al. Epilepsie partielle bénigne et état de mal électroencéphalographique pendant le sommeil. *Rev EEG Neurophysiol* 1978;8:350–3.

Damiano JA, Burgess R, Kivity S, et al. Frequency of *CNKSR2* mutation in the X-linked epilepsy-aphasia spectrum. *Epilepsia* 2017;58(3):e40–3.

de Kovel CGF, Syrbe S, Brilstra EH, et al. Neurodevelopmental disorders caused by de novo variants in *KCNB1* genotypes and phenotypes. *JAMA Neurol* 2017;74(10):1228–36.

de Menezes MS, Warner M, Shurtleff H, Rho J. Clinical characteristics of patients referred to a tertiary center for a history of acute language regression. *Epilepsia* 1998;39:156.

De Negri M. Electrical status epilepticus during sleep (ESES). Different clinical syndromes: towards a unifying view? *Brain Dev* 1997;19:447–51.

De Tiege X, Goldman S, Laureys S, et al. Regional cerebral glucose metabolism in epilepsies with continuous spikes and waves during sleep. *Neurology* 2004;63:853–7.

De Tiege X, Goldman S, Van Bogaert P. Insights into the pathophysiology of psychomotor regression in CSWS syndromes from FDG-PET and EEG-fMRI. *Epilepsia* 2009;50(7):47–50.

De Tiege X, Goldman S, Verheulpen D, Aeby A, Poznanski N, Van Bogaert P. Coexistence of idiopathic rolandic epilepsy and CSWS in two families. *Epilepsia* 2006;47(10):1723–7.

De Tiege X, Harrison S, Laufs H, et al. Impact of interictal epileptic activity on normal brain function in epileptic encephalopathy: an electroencephalography functional magnetic resonance imaging study. *Epilepsy Behav* 2007;11:460–5.

De Tiege X, Ligot N, Goldman S, Poznanski N, de Saint Martin A, van Bogaert P. Metabolic evidence for remote inhibition in epilepsies with continuous spike-waves during sleep. *NeuroImage* 2008;40:802–10.

De Tiege X, Trotta N, Op de Beeck M, et al. Neurophysiological activity underlying altered brain metabolism in epileptic encephalopathies with CSWS. *Epilepsy Res* 2013;105:316–25.

de Vivo L, Bellesi M, Marshall W, et al. Ultrastructural evidence for synaptic scaling across the wake/sleep cycle. *Science* 2017;355:507–10.

de Vivo L, Faraguna U, Nelson AB, et al. Developmental patterns of sleep slow wave activity and synaptic density in adolescent mice. *Sleep* 2014;37:689–700.

de Vries EE, van den Munckhof B, Braun KP, van Royen-Kerkhof A, de Jager W, Jansen FE. Inflammatory mediators in human epilepsy: A systematic review and meta-analysis. *Neurosci Biobehav Rev* 2016;63:177–90.

Depienne C, Gourfinkel-An I, Baulac S, LeGuern E. Genes in infantile epileptic encephalopathies. In: *Jasper's basic mechanisms of the epilepsies*. 4th Ed. Noebels JL, Avoli M, Rogawski MA, Olsen RW, Delgado-Escueta AV. Bethesda (MD), 2012.

Destexhe A, Sejnowski T. *Thalamo-cortical Assemblies*. Oxford UK: Oxford University Press; 2001.

Diekelmann S, Born J. The memory function of sleep. *Nat Rev Neurosci* 2010;11:114–26.

Diering GH, Nirujogi RS, Roth RH, et al. Homer1a drives homeostatic scaling-down of excitatory synapses during sleep. *Science* 2017;355:511–5.

Dimassi S, Labalme A, Lesca G, et al. A subset of genomic alterations detected in rolandic epilepsies contains candidate or known epilepsy genes including *GRIN2A* and *PRRT2*. *Epilepsia* 2014;55(2):370–8.

Doose H, Hahn A, Neubauer BA, Pistohl J, Stephani U. Atypical "benign" partial epilepsy of childhood or pseudo-lennox syndrome. Part II: family study. *Neuropediatrics* 2001;32:9–13.

Dorris L, O'Regan ME, Wilson M, Zuberi SM. Progressive intellectual impairment in children with Encephalopathy related to Status Epilepticus during slow Sleep. In: *Encephalopathy related to Status Epilepticus during slow Sleep: linking epilepsy, sleep disruption and cognitive impairment*. Rubboli G, Tassinari CA, editors. Montrouge: John Libbey Eurotext; 2020. p. 83–92.

Dorris L. Predicting the IQ of young children from early developmental markers. *Eur J Paed Neurol* 2017;21:247.

Downes M, Greenaway R, Jolleff N, et al. Outcome following multiple subpial transection in Landau-Kleffner syndrome and related regression. *Epilepsia* 2015;56(11):1760–6.

Ebus SC, Overvliet GM, Arends JB, Aldenkamp AP. Reading performance in children with rolandic epilepsy correlates with nocturnal epileptiform activity, but not with epileptiform activity while awake. *Epilepsy Behav* 2011;22:518–22.

Endele S, Rosenberger G, Geider K, et al. Mutations in *GRIN2A* and *GRIN2B* encoding regulatory subunits of NMDA receptors cause variable neurodevelopmental phenotypes. *Nat Genet* 2010;42(11):1021–6.

Engel J Jr. International League Against Epilepsy (ILAE). A proposed diagnostic scheme for people with epileptic seizures and with epilepsy: report of the ILAE Task Force on Classification and Terminology. *Epilepsia* 2001;42:796–803.

Engel J Jr. Report of the ILAE classification core group. *Epilepsia* 2006;47:1558–68.

Eriksson K, Kylliainen A, Hirvonen K, Nieminen P, Koivikko M. Visual agnosia in a child with non-lesional occipito-temporal CSWS. *Brain Dev* 2003;25:262–7.

Esser SK, Hill SL, Tononi G. Sleep homeostasis and cortical synchronization: I. Modeling the effects of synaptic strength on sleep slow waves. *Sleep* 2007;30:1617–30.

Farnarier G, Kouna P, Genton P. Amplitude EEG mapping in three cases of CSWS. In: *Continuous spikes and waves during slow sleep, electrical status epilepticus during slow sleep: acquired epileptic aphasia and related conditions*. Beaumanoir M, Bureau M, Deonna T, Mira L, Tassinari CA. London, England: John Libbey & Co; 1995. p. 91–8.

Fattinger S, Schmitt B, Bolsterli Heinzle BK, et al. Impaired slow wave sleep downscaling in patients with infantile spasms. *Eur J Paediatr Neurol* 2015;19:134–42.

Fayad MN, Choueiri R, Mikati M. Landau-Kleffner syndrome: consistent response to repeated intravenous gammaglobulin doses: a case report. *Epilepsia* 1997;38:489–94.

Feinberg I. Schizophrenia: caused by a fault in programmed synaptic elimination during adolescence? *J Psychiatr Res* 1982;17:319–34.

Fejerman N, Caraballo R, Tenembaum SN. Atypical evolutions of benign localization-related epilepsies in children: are they predictable? *Epilepsia* 2000;41:380–90.

Fenn KM, Nusbaum HC, Margoliash D. Consolidation during sleep of perceptual learning of spoken language. *Nature* 2003;425:614–6.

Fernández IS, Chapman KE, Peters JM, et al. The tower of Babel: survey on concepts and terminology in electrical status epilepticus in sleep and continuous spikes and waves during sleep in North America. *Epilepsia* 2013;54:741–50.

Fernández IS, Peters J, Takeoka M, et al. Patients with electrical status epilepticus in sleep share similar clinical features regardless of their focal or generalized sleep potentiation of epileptiform activity. *J Child Neurol* 2013;28:83–9.

Fernández IS, Peters JM, Hadjiloizou S, et al. Clinical staging and electroencephalographic evolution of continuous spikes and waves during sleep. *Epilepsia* 2012;53:1185–95.

Ferri R, Bruni O, Miano S, Smerieri A, Spruyt K, Terzano MG. Inter-rater reliability of sleep cyclic alternating pattern (CAP) scoring and validation of a new computer-assisted CAP scoring method. *Clin Neurophysiol* 2005;116(3):696–707.

Ferrillo F, Beelke M, Nobili L. Sleep EEG synchronization mechanisms and activation of interictal epileptic spikes. *Clin Neurophysiol* 2000;111(2):S65–73.

Filippini M, Arzimanoglou A, Gobbi G. Neuropsychological approaches to epileptic encephalopathies. *Epilepsia* 2013;54:38–44.

Filippini M, Boni A, Giannotta M, Gobbi G. Neuropsychological development in children belonging to BECTS spectrum: long-term effect of epileptiform activity. *Epilepsy Behav* 2013;28:504–11.

Fine AL, Wirrell EC, Wong-Kisiel LC, Nickels KC. Acetazolamide for electrical status epilepticus in slow-wave sleep. *Epilepsia* 2015;56(9):e134–8.

Fisher RS, Acevedo C, Arzimanoglou A, et al. ILAE official report: a practical clinical definition of epilepsy. *Epilepsia* 2014;55:475–82.

Fournier-Del Castillo C, García-Fernández M, Pérez-Jiménez M-Á, et al. Encephalopathy with electrical status epilepticus during sleep: Cognitive and executive improvement after epilepsy surgery. *Seizure* 2014;23:240–3.

Frank MG, Issa NP, Stryker MP. Sleep enhances plasticity in the developing visual cortex. *Neuron* 2001;30:275–87.

Frauscher B, von Ellenrieder N, Dubeau F, Gotman J. EEG desynchronization during phasic REM sleep suppresses interictal epileptic activity in humans. *Epilepsia* 2016;57:879–88.

Frauscher B, von Ellenrieder N, Ferrari-Marinho T, Avoli M, Dubeau F, Gotman J. Facilitation of epileptic activity during sleep is mediated by high amplitude slow waves. *Brain* 2015;138:1629–41.

Gaillard WD, Chiron C, Cross JH, et al. Guidelines for imaging infants and children with recent-onset epilepsy. *Epilepsia* 2009;50:2147–53.

Galanopoulou AS, Bojko A, Lado F, Moshé SL. The spectrum of neuropsychiatric abnormalities associated with electrical status epilepticus in sleep. *Brain Dev* 2000;22(5):279–95.

Gardella E, Cantalupo G, Larsson PG, et al. EEG features in Encephalopathy related to Status Epilepticus during slow Sleep. In: Encephalopathy related to Status Epilepticus during slow Sleep: linking epilepsy, sleep disruption and cognitive impairment. Rubboli G, Tassinari CA, editors. Montrouge: John Libbey Eurotext; 2020. p. 25–36.

Gardella E, Kolmel MS, Terney D, et al. Afternoon NAP vs. all-night sleep EEG for the diagnosis of ESES. *Epilepsia* 2016;57(S2):77.

Gencpinar P, Dundar NO, Tekgul H. Electrical status epilepticus in sleep (ESES)/continuous spikes and waves during slow sleep (CSWS) syndrome in children: An electroclinical evaluation according to the EEG patterns. *Epilepsy Behav* 2016;61:107–11.

Gentry KR, Arnup SJ, Disma N, et al. Enrollment challenges in multi-center, international studies: the example of the GAS trial. *Pediatric Anesthesia* 2019;29(1):51–8.

Gibbs EL, Gibbs FA. Diagnostic and localizing value of electroencephalographic studies in sleep. *Res Publ Assoc Res Nerv Ment Dis* 1947;26:366.

Gibbs SA, Figorilli M, Casaceli G, Proserpio P, Nobili L. Sleep-related hypermotor seizures with a right parietal onset. *J Clin Sleep Med* 2015;11:953–5.

Gibbs SA, Nobili L, Halász P. Interictal epileptiform discharges in sleep and the role of the thalamus in Encephalopathy related to Status Epilepticus during slow Sleep. In: Encephalopathy related to Status Epilepticus during slow Sleep: linking epilepsy, sleep disruption and cognitive impairment. Rubboli G, Tassinari CA, editors. Montrouge: John Libbey Eurotext; 2020. p. 61–7.

Gibbs SA, Proserpio P, Terzaghi M, et al. Sleep-related epileptic behaviors and non-REM-related parasomnias: Insights from stereo-EEG. *Sleep Med Rev* 2016;25:4–20.

Goldberg RF, Ballaban-gil K, Ochoa J, et al. Epileptiform EEG abnormalities in autistic children with a history of language regression. *Epilepsia* 1998;39:156–7.

Gong P, Xue J, Qian P, et al. Scalp-recorded high-frequency oscillations in childhood epileptic encephalopathy with continuous spike-and-wave during sleep with different etiologies. *Brain Dev* 2018;40:299–310.

Gordon N. Cognitive functions and epileptic activity. *Seizure* 2000;9:184–8.

Gotman J, Grova C, Bagshaw A, Kobayashi E, Aghakhani Y, Dubeau F. Generalized epileptic spikes show thalamocortical activation and suspension of the default state of the brain. *PNAS* 2005;102:15236–40.

Grote CL, Van Slyke P, Hoeppner JAB. Language outcome following multiple subpial transection. *Brain* 1999;122:561–6.

Guerrini R, Belmonte A, Genton P. Antiepileptic drug-induced worsening of seizures in children. *Epilepsia* 1998;39(3):S2–10.

Guerrini R, Genton P, Bureau M, et al. Multilobar polymicrogyria, intractable drop attack seizures, and sleep-related electrical status epilepticus. *Neurology* 1998;51(2):504–12.

Guzzetta F, Battaglia D, Veredice C, et al. Early thalamic injury associated with epilepsy and continuous spike-wave during slow sleep. *Epilepsia* 2005;46:889–900.

Haberlandt E, Weger C, Sigl SB, et al. Adrenocorticotropic hormone versus pulsatile dexamethasone in the treatment of infantile epilepsy syndromes. *Pediatr Neurol* 2010;42:21–7.

Hahn A, Pistohl J, Neubauer BA, Stephani U. Atypical "benign" partial epilepsy or pseudo-Lennox syndrome. Part I: symptomatology and long-term prognosis. *Neuropediatrics* 2001;32:1–8.

Halasz P, Hegyi M, Siegler Z, Fogarasi A. Encephalopathy with electrical status epilepticus in slow wave sleep - a review with an emphasis on regional (perisylvian) aspects. *J Epileptol* 2014;22:107–23.

Halasz P, Kelemen A, Clemens B, et al. The perisylvian epileptic network. A unifying concept. *Ideggyógy Szle* 2005;58:21–31.

Halasz P, Kelemen A, Szűcs A. The role of NREM sleep microarousals in absence epilepsy and in nocturnal frontal lobe epilepsy. *Epilepsy Res* 2013;107:9–19.

Halasz P, Terzano M, Parrino L, Bodizs R. The nature of arousal in sleep. *J Sleep Res* 2004;13:1–23.

Helbig I, Mefford HC, Sharp AJ, et al. 15q13.3 microdeletions increase risk of idiopathic generalized epilepsy. *Nat Genet* 2009;41(2):160–2.

Herman ST, Walczak TS, Bazil CW. Distribution of partial seizures during the sleep-wake cycle: differences by seizure onset site. *Neurology* 2001;56:1453–9.

Hirata A, Castro-Alamancos MA. Neocortex network activation and deactivation states controlled by the thalamus. *J Neurophysiol* 2010;103:1147–57.

Hirsch E, Caraballo R, Dalla Bernardina B, Loddenkemper T, Zuberi SM. Encephalopathy related to Status Epilepticus during slow Sleep : from concepts to terminology. In: Encephalopathy related to Status Epilepticus during slow Sleep: linking epilepsy, sleep disruption and cognitive impairment. Rubboli G, Tassinari CA, editors. Montrouge: John Libbey Eurotext; 2020. p. 7–16.

Hirsch E, Maquet P, Metz-Lutz MN, et al. The eponym 'Landau-Kleffner syndrome' should not be restricted to childhood-acquired aphasia with epilepsy. In: *Continuous spikes and waves during slow sleep*. Beaumanoir A, Bureau T, Deonna T, Mira L, Tassinari CA. Oxford: John Libbey &Company Ltd; 1995. p. 57–62.

Hirsch E, Marescaux C, Maquet P, et al. Landau-Kleffner syndrome: a clinical and EEG study of five cases. *Epilepsia* 1990;31:756–67.

Hirsch E, Valenti MP, Rudolph G, et al. Landau-Kleffner syndrome is not an eponymic badge of ignorance. *Epilepsy Res* 2006;70(1):S239–47.

Hoel E, Albantakis L, Cirelli C, Tononi G. Synaptic refinement during development and its effect on slow wave activity - a computational study. *J Neurophysiol* 2016;115:199–213.

Holmes GL, Lenck-Santini P. Role of interictal epileptiform abnormalities in cognitive impairment. *Epilepsy Behav* 2006;8:504–15.

Hommet C, Billard C, Motte J, et al. Cognitive function in adolescents and young adults in complete remission from benign childhood epilepsy with centro-temporal spikes. *Epileptic Disord* 2001;3(4):207–16.

Huber R, Ghilardi MF, Massimini M, et al. Arm immobilization causes cortical plastic changes and locally decreases sleep slow wave activity. *Nat Neurosci* 2006;9:1169–76.

Huber R, Ghilardi MF, Massimini M, Tononi G. Local sleep and learning. *Nature* 2004;430:78–81.

Hughes JR. A review of the relationships between Landau-Kleffner syndrome, electrical status epilepticus during sleep and continuous spike-waves during sleep. *Epilepsy Behav* 2011;20(2):247–53.

Huttenlocher PR, Dabholkar AS. Regional differences in synaptogenesis in human cerebral cortex. *J Comp Neurol* 1997;387:167–78.

Huttenlocher PR. Synaptic density in human frontal cortex - developmental change and effects of aging. *Brain Res* 1979;163:195–205.

Iber C, Ancoli-Israel S, Chesson AL, Quan SF. *The AASM manual for the scoring of sleep and associated events: rules, terminology and technical specification*. Westchester, IL: AASM; 2007.

Inutsuka M, Kobayashi K, Oka M, Hattori J, Ohtsuka Y. Treatment of epilepsy with electrical status epilepticus during slow sleep and its related disorders. *Brain Dev* 2006;28:281–6.

Issa NP. Neurobiology of continuous spike-wave in slowwave sleep and Landau-Kleffner syndromes. *Ped Neurol* 2014;51:287–96.

Japaridze N, Muthuraman M, Dierck C, et al. Neuronal networks in epileptic encephalopathies with CSWS. *Epilepsia* 2016;57:1245–55.

Jehi L, Wyllie E, Devinsky O. Epileptic encephalopathies: optimizing control and developmental outcome. *Epilepsia* 2015;56:1486–9.

Jeong A, Strahle J, Vellimana AK, Limbrick DD Jr, Smyth MD, Bertrand M. Hemispherotomy in children with electrical status epilepticus of sleep. *J Neurosurg Pediatr* 2017;19:56–62.

Jha SK, Jones BE, Coleman T, et al. Sleep-dependent plasticity requires cortical activity. *J Neurosci* 2005;25:9266–74.

Joshi CN, Chapman KE, Bear JJ, Wilson SB, Walleigh DJ, Scheuer ML. Semiautomated spike detection software Persyst 13 is noninferior to human readers when calculating the Spike-Wave Index in Electrical Status Epilepticus in Sleep. *J Clin Neurophysiol* 2018;35:370–4.

Kadish NE, Baumann M, Pietz J, Schubert-Bast S, Reuner G. Validation of a screening tool for attention and executive functions (EpiTrack Junior) in children and adolescents with absence epilepsy. *Epilepsy Behav* 2013;29:96–102.

Kallay C, Mayor-Dubois C, Maeder-Ingvar M, et al. Reversible acquired epileptic frontal syndrome and CSWS suppression in a child with congenital hemiparesis treated by hemispherotomy. *Eur J Paediatr Neurol* 2009;13:430–8.

Kanemura H, Sugita K, Aihara M. Prefrontal lobe growth in a patient with continuous spike-waves during slow sleep. *Neuropediatrics* 2009;40:192–4.

Kelemen A, Barsi P, Gyorsok Z, Sarac J, Szucs A, Halasz P. Thalamic lesion and epilepsy with generalized seizures. ESES and spike-wave paroxysms-report of three cases. *Seizure* 2006;15:454–8.

Kellerman K. Recurrent aphasia with subclinical bioelectric status epilepticus during sleep. *Eur J Pediatr* 1978;128:207–12.

Kelley SA, Kossoff EH. How effective is the ketogenic diet for electrical status epilepticus of sleep? *Epilepsy Res* 2016;127:339–43.

Kleffner FR, Landau WM. The Landau-Kleffner syndrome. *Epilepsia* 2009;50(7):3.

Kobayashi K, Nishibayashi N, Ohtsuka Y, Oka E, Ohtahara S. Epilepsy with electrical status epilepticus during slow sleep and secondary bilateral synchrony. *Epilepsia* 1994;35:1097–103.

Kobayashi K, Watanabe Y, Inoue T, Oka M, Yoshinaga H, Ohtsuka Y. Scalp-recorded high-frequency oscillations in childhood sleep-induced electrical status epilepticus. *Epilepsia* 2010;51:2190–4.

Kobayashi K, Yoshinaga H, Toda Y, Inoue T, Oka M, Ohtsuka Y. High-frequency oscillations in idiopathic partial epilepsy of childhood. *Epilepsia* 2011;52:1812–9.

Kramer U, Sagi L, Goldberg-Stern H, Zelnik N, Nissenkorn A, Ben-Zeev B. Clinical spectrum and medical treatment of children with electrical status epilepticus in sleep (ESES). *Epilepsia* 2009;50:1517–24.

Kuki I, Kawawaki H, Okazaki S, Ikeda H, Tomiwa K. Epileptic encephalopathy with continuous spikes and waves in the occipito-temporal region during slow-wave sleep in two patients with acquired Kanji dysgraphia. *Epileptic Disord* 2014;16:540–5.

Kurth S, Jenni OG, Riedner BA, et al. Characteristics of sleep slow waves in children and adolescents. *Sleep* 2010;33:475–80.

Kurth S, Ringli M, Geiger A, LeBourgeois M, Jenni OG, Huber R. Mapping of cortical activity in the first two decades of life: a high-density sleep electroencephalogram study. *J Neurosci* 2010;30:13211–9.

Kurth S, Ringli M, Lebourgeois MK, et al. Mapping the electrophysiological marker of sleep depth reveals skill maturation in children and adolescents. *NeuroImage* 2012;63:959–65.

Lai CS, Fisher SE, Hurst JA, Vargha-Khadem F, Monaco AP. A forkhead-domain gene is mutated in a severe speech and language disorder. *Nature* 2001;413(6855):519–23.

Lal D, Reinthaler EM, Altmuller J, et al. *RBFOX1* and *RBFOX3* mutations in rolandic epilepsy. *PLoS One* 2013;8(9). e73323.

Lal D, Reinthaler EM, Schubert J, et al. *DEPDC5* mutations in genetic focal epilepsies of childhood. *Ann Neurol* 2014;75(5):788–92.

Landau WM, Kleffner FR. Syndrome of acquired aphasia with convulsive disorder in children. *Neurology* 1957;7(8):523–30.

Larrieu J, Lagueny A, Ferrer X, Jullien J. Épilepsie avec décharges continues au cours du sommeil lent. Guérison sous clobazam. *Rev EEG Nuerophysiol Clin* 1986;16:383–94.

Larsson PG, Bakke KA, Bjørnæs H, et al. The effect of levetiracetam on focal nocturnal epileptiform activity during sleep – A placebo-controlled double-blind cross-over study. *Epilepsy Behav* 2012;24:44–8.

Larsson PG, Eeg-Olofsson O, Michel CM, Seeck M, Lantz G. Decrease in propagation of interictal epileptiform activity after introduction of levetiracetam visualized with electric source imaging. *Brain Topogr* 2010;23:269–78.

Larsson PG, Evsiukova T, Brockmeier F, Ramm-Pettersen A, Eeg-Olofsson O. Do sleep-deprived EEG recordings reflect spike index as found in full-night EEG recordings? *Epilepsy Behav* 2010;19:348–51.

Larsson PG, Wilson J, Eeg-Olofsson O. A new method for quantification and assessment of epileptiform activity in EEG with special reference to focal nocturnal epileptiform activity. *Brain Topogr* 2009;22:52–9.

Leal A, Calado E, Vieira JP, et al. Anatomical and physiological basis of continuous spike-wave of sleep syndrome after early thalamic lesions. *Epilepsy Behav* 2018;78:243–55.

Lee HY, Huang Y, Bruneau N, et al. Mutations in the novel protein *PRRT2* cause paroxysmal kinesigenic dyskinesia with infantile convulsions. *Cell Rep* 2012;1(1):2–12.

Lehtimaki KA, Liimatainen S, Peltola J, et al. The serum level of interleukin-6 in patients with intellectual disability and refractory epilepsy. *Epilepsy Res* 2011;95:184–7.

Leite JP, Neder L, Arisi GM, et al. Plasticity, synaptic strength, and epilepsy: what can we learn from ultrastructural data? *Epilepsia* 2005;46(5):134–41.

Lemke JR, Lal D, Reinthaler EM, et al. Mutations in GRIN2A cause idiopathic focal epilepsy with rolandic spikes. *Nat Genet* 2013;45(9):1067–72.

Lerman P, Lerman-Sagie T, Kivity S. Effect of early corticosteroid therapy for Landau-Kleffner syndrome. *Dev Med Child Neurol* 1991;33:257–60.

Lesca G, Rudolf G, Bruneau N, et al. GRIN2A mutations in acquired epileptic aphasia and related childhood focal epilepsies and encephalopathies with speech and language dysfunction. *Nat Genet* 2013;45(9):1061–6.

Lesca G, Rudolf G, Labalme A, et al. Epileptic encephalopathies of the Landau-Kleffner and continuous spike and waves during slow-wave sleep types: genomic dissection makes the link with autism. *Epilepsia* 2012;53(9):1526–38.

Ligot N, Archambaud F, Trotta N, et al. Default mode network hypometabolism in epileptic encephalopathies with CSWS. *Epilepsy Res* 2014;108:861–71.

Lim ET, Raychaudhuri S, Sanders SJ, et al. Rare complete knockouts in humans: population distribution and significant role in autism spectrum disorders. *Neuron* 2013;77(2):235–42.

Liu J, Lee HJ, Weitz AJ, et al. Frequency-selective control of cortical and subcortical networks by central thalamus. *Elife* 2015;4. e09215.

Liu X, Somel M, Tang L, et al. Extension of cortical synaptic development distinguishes humans from chimpanzees and macaques. *Genome Res* 2012;22:611–22.

Liukkonen E, Kantola-Sorsa E, Paetau R, Gaily E, Peltola M. Granström M-L. Long-term outcome of 32 children with encephalopathy with status epilepticus during sleep, or ESES syndrome. *Epilepsia* 2010;51:2023–32.

Loddenkemper T, Cosmo G, Kotagal P, et al. Epilepsy surgery in children with electrical status epilepticus in sleep. *Neurosurgery* 2009;64:328–37.

Loddenkemper T, Sanchez Fernandez I, Peters M. Continuous spike and waves during sleep and electrical status epilepticus in sleep. *J Clin Neurophysiol* 2011;28:154–64.

Malow BA, Lin X, Kushwaha R, Aldrich MS. Interictal spiking increases with sleep depth in temporal lobe epilepsy. *Epilepsia* 1998;39:1309.

Maquet P, Hirsch E, Metz-Lutz MN, et al. Regional cerebral glucose metabolism in children with deterioration of one or more cognitive functions and continuous spike-and-wave discharges during sleep. *Brain* 1995;118:1497–520.

Maret S, Faraguna U, Nelson AB, Cirelli C, Tononi G. Sleep and waking modulate spine turnover in the adolescent mouse cortex. *Nat Neurosci* 2011;14:1418–20.

Margari L, Buttiglione M, Legrottaglie AR, Presicci A, Craig F, Curatolo P. Neuropsychiatric impairment in children with Continuous Spikes and Waves during slow Sleep: A long-term follow-up study. *Epilepsy Behav* 2012;25(4):558–62.

Marini C, Romoli M, Parrini E, et al. Clinical features and outcome of 6 new patients carrying de novo KCNB1 gene mutations. *Neurol Genet* 2017;3(6):e206.

Masnada S, Hedrich UBS, Gardella E, et al. Clinical spectrum and genotype-phenotype associations of KCNA2-related encephalopathies. *Brain* 2017;140(9):2337–54.

Massa R, de Saint-Martin A, Carcangiu R, et al. EEG criteria predictive of complicated evolution in idiopathic rolandic epilepsy. *Neurology* 2001;57(6):1071–9.

Massa R, de Saint-Martin A, Hirsch E, et al. Landau-Kleffner syndrome: sleep EEG characteristics at onset. *Clin Neurophysiol* 2000;111(S2):S87–93.

Mathieu ML, de Bellescize J, Till M, et al. Electrical status epilepticus in sleep, a constitutive feature of Christianson syndrome? *Eur J Paediatr Neurol* 2018;(17):31980–3.

Meeren H, van Luijtelaar G, Lopes da Silva F, Coenen A. Evolving concepts on the pathophysiology of absence seizures: the cortical focus theory. *Arch Neurol* 2005;62:371–6.

Mefford HC, Muhle H, Ostertag P, et al. Genome-wide copy number variation in epilepsy: novel susceptibility loci in idiopathic generalized and focal epilepsies. *PLoS Genet* 2010;6(5).

Mikati MA, Saab R, Fayad MN, Choueiri RN. Efficacy of intravenous immunoglobulin in Landau-Kleffner syndrome. *Pediatr Neurol* 2002;26:298–300.

Mirandola L, Cantalupo G, Vaudano AE, et al. Centrotemporal spikes during NREM sleep: The promoting action of thalamus revealed by simultaneous EEG and fMRI coregistration. *Epilepsy Behav Case Rep* 2013;1:106–9.

Moeller F, Stephani U, Siniatchkin M. Simultaneous EEG and fMRI recordings (EEG-fMRI) in children with epilepsy. *Epilepsia* 2013;54:971–82.

Monteiro JP, Roulet-Perez E, Davidoff V, Deonna T. Primary neonatal thalamic haemorrhage and epilepsy with continuous spike-wave during sleep: a longitudinal follow-up of a possible significant relation. *Eur J Paediatr Neurol* 2001;5:41–7.

Morikawa T, Masakazu S, Watanabe M. Long-term outcome of CSWS syndrome. In: *Continuous spikes and waves during slow sleep*. Beaumanoir A, Bureau T, Deonna T, Mira L, Tassinari CA. Oxford: John Libbey &Company Ltd; 1995. p. 27–36.

Morikawa T, Seino M, Osawa T, Yagi K. Five children with continuous spike-waves discharges during sleep. In: *Epileptic syndromes in infancy, childhood and adolescence*. Roger J, Dravet C, Bureau M, Dreifuss FE, Wolf P. London: John Libbey; 1985. p. 205–12.

Morikawa T, Seino M, Watanabe M. Continuous spikes and waves during slow sleep. Electrical status epilepticus during slow sleep. In: *Epileptic syndromes in infancy, childhood and adolescence*. 5th Ed. Beaumanoir A, et al. London: John Libbey; 1995. p. 27–36.

Morikawa T, Seino M, Watanabe Y, Watanabe M, Yagi K. Clinical relevance of continuous spike-waves during slow wave sleep. In: *Advances in epileptology*. Manelis S, Bental E, Loeber JN, Dreifuss FE. New York: Raven Press; 1989. p. 359–63.

Morita DA, Glauser TA, Modi AC. Development and validation of the pediatric side effects questionnaire. *Neurology* 2012;79:1252–8.

Morrell F, Whisler WW, Smith MC, *et al*. Landau-Kleffner syndrome. Treatment with subpial intracortical transection. *Brain* 1995;118:1529–46.

Mouridsen SE, Videbaek C, Sogaard H, Andersen AR. Regional cerebral blood-flow measured by HMPAO and SPECT in a 5-year old boy with Landau-Kleffner syndrome. *Neuropediatrics* 1993;24:47–50.

Nelson AB, Faraguna U, Zoltan JT, Tononi G, Cirelli C. Sleep patterns and homeostatic mechanisms in adolescent mice. *Brain Sci* 2013;3:318–43.

Neubauer BA, Fiedler B, Himmelein B, *et al*. Centrotemporal spikes in families with rolandic epilepsy: linkage to chromosome 15q14. *Neurology* 1998;51(6):1608–12.

Neville BGR, Burch V, Cass H, Lees J. Motor disorders in Landau-Kleffner syndrome (LKS). *Epilepsia* 1998;39(6):123.

Nieuwenhuis L, Nicolai J. The pathophysiological mechanisms of cognitive and behavioral disturbances in children with Landau-Kleffner syndrome or epilepsy with continuous spike-and-waves during slow-wave sleep. *Seizure* 2006;15(4):249–58.

Nikanorova M, Miranda MJ, Atkins M, Sahlholdt L. Ketogenic diet in the treatment of refractory continuous spikes and waves during slow sleep. *Epilepsia* 2009;50:1127–31.

Nir Y, Staba RJ, Andrillon T, *et al*. Regional slow waves and spindles in human sleep. *Neuron* 2011;70:153–69.

Nobili L, Baglietto MG, Beelke M, *et al*. Distribution of epileptiform discharges during nREM sleep in the CSWSS syndrome: relationship with sigma and delta activities. *Epilepsy Res* 2001;44:119–28.

Nobili L, Baglietto MG, Beelke M, *et al*. Spindles-inducing mechanism modulates sleep activation of interictal epileptiform discharges in the Landau-Kleffner syndrome. *Epilepsia* 2000;41:201–6.

Nobili L, Ferrillo F, Baglietto MG, *et al*. Relationship of sleep interictal epileptiform discharges to sigma activity (12-16 Hz) in benign epilepsy of childhood with rolandic spikes. *Clin Neurophysiol* 1999;110:39–46.

Nonclercq A, Foulon M, Verheulpen D, *et al*. Cluster-based spike detection algorithm adapts to interpatient and intrapatient variation in spike morphology. *J Neurosci Methods* 2012;210(2):259–65.

Nonclercq A, Foulon M, Verheulpen D, *et al*. Spike detection algorithm automatically adapted to individual patients applied to spike-and-wave percentage quantification. *Neurophysiol Clin* 2009;39(2):123–31.

Olini N, Kurth S, Huber R. The effects of caffeine on sleep and maturational markers in the rat. *PLoS ONE* 2013;8. e72539.

Paetau R, Granstrom ML, Blomstedt G, Jousmäki V, Korkman M, Liukkone E. Magnetoencephalography in presurgical evaluation of children with the Landau-Kleffner syndrome. *Epilepsia* 1999;40:326–35.

Panayiotopoulos CP, Micheal M, Sanders S, Valeta T, Koutroumanidis M. Benign childhood focal epilepsies: assessment of established and newly recognized syndromes. *Brain* 2008;131:2264–86.

Panayiotopoulos CP. Epileptic encephalopathies in infancy and early childhood in which the epileptiform abnormalities may contribute to progressive dysfunction. In: *The epilepsies Seizures, syndromes and management.* Panayiotopoulos CP. Oxford: Bladon Medical Publishing; 2005. p. 137–206.

Panayiotopoulos CP. Severe syndromes of mainly linguistic and neuropsychological deficits, seizures or both and marked EEG abnormalities from the Rolandic and neighbouring regions. In: *Benign childhood partial seizures and related epileptic syndromes.* Panayiotopoulos CP. London: John Libbey; 1999. p. 337–60.

Parisi P, Bruni O, Pia Villa M, *et al.* The relationship between sleep and epilepsy: the effect on cognitive functioning in children. *Dev Med Child Neurol* 2010;52:805–10.

Parlatini V, Radua J, Dell'Acqua F, *et al.* Functional segregation and integration within fronto-parietal networks. *NeuroImage* 2017;146:367–75.

Parrino L, Halasz P, Tassinari CA, Terzano MG. CAP, epilepsy and motor events during sleep: the unifying role of arousal. *Sleep Med Rev* 2006;10:267–85.

Patry G, Lyagoubi S, Tassinari CA. Subclinical "electrical status epilepticus" induced by sleep in children. A clinical and electroencephalographic study of six cases. *Arch Neurol* 1971;24:242–52.

Pavlidis E, Rubboli G, Nikanorova M, Kolmel MS, Gardella E. Encephalopathy with status epilepticus during sleep (ESES) induced by oxcarbazepine in idiopathic focal epilepsy in childhood. *Funct Neurol* 2015;8:1–3.

Paz JT, Christian CA, Parada I, Prince DA, Huguenard JR. Focal cortical infarcts alter intrinsic excitability and synaptic excitation in the reticular thalamic nucleus. *J Neurosci* 2010;30:5465–79.

Péchadre JC, Sauvezie B, Osier C, Gibert J. The treatment of epileptic encephalopathies with gamma globulin in children (author's transl). *Rev Electroencephalogr Neurophysiol Clin* 1977;7:443–7.

Peltola M, Liukkonen E, Granström M, *et al.* The effect of surgery in encephalopathy with status epilepticus during sleep. *Epilepsia* 2011;52:602–9.

Peltola ME, Palmu K, Liukkonen E, Gaily E, Vanhatalo S. Semiautomatic quantification of spiking in patients with continuous spikes and waves in sleep: sensitivity to settings and correspondence to visual assessment. *Clin Neurophysiol* 2012;123(7):1284–90.

Peltola ME, Sairanen V, Gaily E, Vanhatalo S. Measuring spike strength in patients with continuous spikes and waves during sleep: comparison of methods for prospective use as a clinical index. *Clin Neurophysiol* 2014;125:1639–46.

Pera M, Brazzo D, Altieri N, Balottin U, Veggiotti P. Long-term evolution of neuropsychological competences in encephalopathy with status epilepticus during sleep: A variable prognosis. *Epilepsia* 2013;54:77–85.

Petanjek Z, Judaš M, Šimic G, *et al.* Extraordinary neoteny of synaptic spines in the human prefrontal cortex. *PNAS* 2011;108:13281–6.

Pierson TM, Yuan H, Marsh ED, *et al.* GRIN2A mutation and early-onset epileptic encephalopathy: personalized therapy with memantine. *Ann Clin Transl Neurol* 2014;1(3):190–8.

Praline J, Hommet C, Barthez MA, *et al.* Outcome at adulthood of the continuous spike-waves during slow sleep and Landau Kleffner syndromes. *Epilepsia* 2003;44:1434–40.

Qian P, Li H, Xue J, Yang Z. Scalp-recorded high-frequency oscillations in atypical benign partial epilepsy. *Clin Neurophysiol* 2016;127:3306–13.

Raichle ME, MacLeod AM, Snyder AZ, Powers WJ, Gusnard DA, Shulman GL. A default mode of brain function. *PNAS* 2001;98:676–82.

Raichle ME, Mintun MA. Brain work and brain imaging. *Ann Rev Neurosci* 2006;29:449–76.

Rakic P, Bourgeois JP, Goldman-Rakic PS. Synaptic development of the cerebral cortex: implications for learning, memory, and mental illness. *Prog Brain Res* 1994;102:227–43.

Rechtschaffen A, Kales A. *A Manual of standardized terminology, techniques and scoring system for sleep stages of human subjects.* Washington DC: Washington Public Health Service, US Government Printing Office; 1968.

Reinthaler EM, Dejanovic B, Lal D, Semtner M, Merkler Y, Reinhold A. Rare variants in γ-aminobutyric acid type A receptor genes in rolandic epilepsy and related syndromes. *Ann Neurol* 2015;77(6):972–86.

Reinthaler EM, Lal D, Jurkowski W, et al. Analysis of *ELP4*, *SRPX2*, and interacting genes in typical and atypical rolandic epilepsy. *Epilepsia* 2014;55(8):e89–93.

Reinthaler EM, Lal D, Lebon S, et al. 16p11.2 600 kb Duplications confer risk for typical and atypical Rolandic epilepsy. *Hum Mol Genet* 2014;23(22):6069–80.

Reutlinger C, Helbig I, Gawelczyk B, et al. Deletions in 16p13 including *GRIN2A* in patients with intellectual disability, various dysmorphic features, and seizure disorders of the rolandic region. *Epilepsia* 2010;51(9):1870–3.

Reyes G, Flesler S, Armeno M, et al. Ketogenic diet in patients with epileptic encephalopathy with electrical status epilepticus during slow sleep. *Epilepsy Res* 2015;113:126–31.

Reynolds CM, Short MA, Gradisar M. Sleep spindles and cognitive performance across adolescence: a meta-analytic review. *J Adolesc* 2018;66:55–70.

Riedner BA, Vyazovskiy VV, Huber R, et al. Sleep homeostasis and cortical synchronization: III. A high-density EEG study of sleep slow waves in humans. *Sleep* 2007;30:1643–57.

Roll P, Rudolf G, Pereira S, et al. *SRPX2* mutations in disorders of language cortex and cognition. *Hum Mol Genet* 2006;15(7):1195–207.

Roll P, Vernes SC, Bruneau N, et al. Molecular networks implicated in speech-related disorders: *FOXP2* regulates the *SRPX2/uPAR* complex. *Hum Mol Genet* 2010;19(24):4848–60.

Romcy-Pereira RN, Leite JP, Garcia-Cairasco N. Synaptic plasticity along the sleep-wake cycle: implications for epilepsy. *Epilepsy Behav* 2009;14:47–53.

Roulet-Perez E, Davidoff V, Despland PA, Deonna T. Mental and behavioural deterioration of children with epilepsy and CSWS: acquired epileptic frontal syndrome. *Dev Med Child Neurol* 1993;35(8):661–74.

Roulet-Perez E, Davidoff V, Mayor-Dubois C, et al. Impact of severe epilepsy on development: recovery potential after successful early epilepsy surgery. *Epilepsia* 2010;51:1266–76.

Rousselle C, Revol M. Relations between cognitive functions and continuous spikes and waves during slow sleep. In: Continuous spikes and waves during slow sleep. Electrical status epilepticus during slow sleep: acquired epileptic aphasia and related conditions. Beaumanoir A, Bureau M, Deonna T, et al. London: John Libbey; 1995. p. 123–33.

Rubboli G, Huber R, Tononi G, Tassinari CA. Encephalopathy related to Status Epilepticus during slow Sleep: a link with sleep homeostasis? In: Encephalopathy related to Status Epilepticus during slow Sleep: linking epilepsy, sleep disruption and cognitive impairment. Rubboli G, Tassinari CA, editors. Montrouge: John Libbey Eurotext; 2020. p. 69–76.

Rudolf G, Valenti MP, Hirsch E, Szepetowski P. From rolandic epilepsy to continuous spike-and-waves during sleep and Landau-Kleffner syndromes: insights into possible genetic factors. *Epilepsia* 2009;50(7):25–8.

Ryan SG. Partial epilepsy: chinks in the armour. *Nat Genet* 1995;10(1):4–6.

Salmi M, Bolbos R, Bauer S, Minlebaev M, Burnashev N, Szepetowski P. Transient microstructural brain anomalies and epileptiform discharges in mice defective for epilepsy and language-related NMDA receptor subunit gene Grin2a. *Epilepsia* 2018;59(10):1919–30.

Salmi M, Bruneau N, Cillario J, et al. Tubacin prevents neuronal migration defects and epileptic activity caused by rat Srpx2 silencing in utero. *Brain* 2013;136(8):2457–73.

Saltik S, Uluduz D, Cokar O, Demirbilek V, Dervent A. A clinical and EEG study on idiopathic partial epilepsies with evolution into ESES spectrum disorders. *Epilepsia* 2005;46:524–33.

Sammaritano M, Gigli JL, Gotman J. Interictal spiking during wakefulness and sleep and the localization of foci in temporal lobe epilepsy. *Neurology* 1991;41:290–7.

Sanchez Fernandez I, Chapman KE, Peters JM, et al. The tower of Babel: survey on concepts and terminology in electrical status epilepticus in sleep and continuous spikes and waves during sleep in North America. *Epilepsia* 2013;54:741–50.

Sanchez Fernandez I, Chapman KE, Peters JM, Harini C, Rotenberg A, Loddenkemper T. Continuous spikes and waves during sleep: electroclinical presentation and suggestions for management. *Epilepsy Res Treat* 2013;2013:583531.

Sanchez Fernandez I, Hadjiloizou S, Eksioglu Y. Short-term response of sleep-potentiated spiking to high-dose diazepam in electric status epilepticus during sleep. *Pediatr Neurol* 2012;46:312–8.

Sanchez Fernandez I, Loddenkemper T, Galanopoulou AS, Moshe SL. Should epileptiform discharges be treated? *Epilepsia* 2015;56:1492–504.

Sanchez Fernandez I, Loddenkemper T, Peters JM, Kothare SV. Electrical status epilepticus in sleep: clinical presentation and pathophysiology. *Pediatric Neurol* 2012;47:390–410.

Sanchez Fernandez I, Peters JM, Akhondi-Asl A, Klehm J, Warfield SK, Loddenkemper T. Reduced thalamic volume in patients with electrical status epilepticus in sleep. *Epilepsy Res* 2017;130:74–80.

Sánchez Fernández I, Peters JM, Hadjiloizou S, et al. Clinical staging and electroencephalographic evolution of continuous spikes and waves during sleep. *Epilepsia* 2012;53:1185–95.

Sanchez Fernandez I, Takeoka M, Tas E, et al. Early thalamic lesions in patients with sleep-potentiated epileptiform activity. *Neurology* 2012;78:1721–7.

Scheffer I, Berkovic S, Capovilla G, et al. ILAE classification of the epilepsies: Position paper of the ILAE Commission for Classification and Terminology. *Epilepsia* 2017;58:512–21.

Scheffer IE, Jones L, Pozzebon M, Howell RA, Saling MM, Berkovic SF. Autosomal dominant rolandic epilepsy and speech dyspraxia: a new syndrome with anticipation. *Ann Neurol* 1995;38(4):633–42.

Scheltens-de Boer M. Guidelines for EEG in encephalopathy related to ESES/CSWS in children. *Epilepsia* 2009;50(S7):13–7.

Scherg M, Ille N, Weckesser D, et al. Fast evaluation of interictal spikes in long-term EEG by hyper-clustering. *Epilepsia* 2012;53(7):1196–204.

Scholtes FB, Hendriks MP, Renier WO. Cognitive deterioration and electrical status epilepticus during slow sleep. *Epilepsy Behav* 2005;6(2):167–73.

Schreiner T, Rasch B. The beneficial role of memory reactivation for language learning during sleep: A review. *Brain Lang* 2017;167:94–105.

Sculier C, Tilmant AS, De Tiège X, et al. Acquired epileptic opercular syndrome related to a heterozygous deleterious substitution in GRIN2A. *Epileptic Disord* 2017;19(3):345–50.

Seegmuller C, Deonna T, Dubois CM, et al. Long-term outcome after cognitive and behavioral regression in nonlesional epilepsy with continuous spike-waves during slow-wave sleep. *Epilepsia* 2012;53:1067–76.

Seri S, Thai JN, Brazzo D, Pisani F, Cerquiglini A. Neurophysiology of CSWS-associated cognitive dysfunction. *Epilepsia* 2009;50(7):33–6.

Shirashi H, Haginoya K, Nakagawa E, et al. Magnetoencephalography localizing spike sources of atypical binighn partial epilepsy. *Brain Dev* 2014;36:21–7.

Sia GM, Clem RL, Huganir RL. The human language-associated gene *SRPX2* regulates synapse formation and vocalization in mice. *Science* 2013;342(6161):987–91.

Sibarov DA, Bruneau N, Antonov SM, Szepetowski P, Burnashev N, Giniatullin R. Functional properties of human NMDA receptors associated with epilepsy-related mutations of GluN2A subunit. *Front Cell Neurosci* 2017;11:155.

Sinclair DB, Snyder TJ. Corticosteroids for the treatment of Landau-kleffner syndrome and continuous spike-wave discharge during sleep. *Pediatr Neurol* 2005;32:300–6.

Siniatchkin M, Groening K, Moehring J, et al. Neuronal networks in children with continuous spikes and waves during slow sleep. *Brain* 2010;133:2798–813.

Sobel DF, Aung M, Otsubo H, Smith MC. Magnetoencephalography in children with Landau-Kleffner syndrome and acquired epileptic aphasia. *Am J Neuroradiol* 2000;21:301–7.

Solomon GE, Carson D, Pavalkis S, Fraser R, Labar D, Intracranial EEG. monitoring in Landau-Kleffner syndrome associated with left temporal lobe astrocytoma. *Epilepsia* 1993;34:557–60.

Soprano AM, Garcia EF, Caraballo R, Fejerman N. Acquired epileptic aphasia: neuropsychologic follow-up of 12 patients. *Pediatr Neurol* 1994;11(3):230–5.

Steinlein OK, Mulley JC, Propping P, et al. A missense mutation in the neuronal nicotinic acetylcholine receptor alpha 4 subunit is associated with autosomal dominant nocturnal frontal lobe epilepsy. *Nat Genet* 1995;11(2):201–3.

Steriade M, Contreras D. Relations between cortical and thalamic cellular events during transition from sleep patterns to paroxysmal activity. *J Neurosci* 1995;15:623–42.

Steriade M, Nunez A, Amzica F. A novel slow (<1 Hz) oscillations of neocortical neurons in vivos: depolarizing and hyperpolarizing components. *J Neurosci* 1993;13:3252–65.

Stickgold R, James L, Hobson JA. Visual discrimination learning requires sleep after training. *Nat Neurosci* 2000;3:1237–8.

Strehlow V, Heyne HO, Lemke JR. The spectrum of GRIN2Aassociated disorders. *Epileptologie* 2015;32:147–51.

Strug LJ, Clarke T, Chiang T, et al. Centrotemporal sharpwave EEG trait in rolandic epilepsy maps to Elongator Protein Complex 4 (ELP4). Eur J Hum Genet 2009;17(9):1171–81.

Swanger SA, Chen W, Wells G, et al. Mechanistic insight into NMDA receptor dysregulation by rare variants in the GluN2A and GluN2B agonist binding domains. Am J Hum Genet 2016;99(6): 1261–80.

Syrbe S, Hedrich UB, Riesch E, et al. De novo loss or gain-of-function mutations in KCNA2 cause epileptic encephalopathy. Nat Genet 2015;47(4):393–9.

Tassinari CA, Bureau M, Dravet C, Dalla Bernardina B, Roger J. Epilepsy with continuous spikes and waves during slow sleep-otherwise described as ESES (epilepsy with electrical status epilepticus during slow sleep). In: *Epileptic syndromes in infancy, childhood and adolescence*. Roger J, Dravet C, Bureau M, Dreifuss FE, Wolf P. London: John Libbey; 1985. p. 194–204.

Tassinari CA, Cantalupo G, Dalla Bernardina B, et al. Encephalopathy related to status epilepticus during slow wave sleep (ESES) including Landau-Kleffner. In: *Epileptic syndromes in infancy, childhood and adolescence*. Bureau M, Genton P, Dravet C, Delgado-Escueta AV, Guerrini R, Tassinari CA, Thomas P, Wolf P, editors. Montrouge: Jihn LIbbey; 2019. p. 261–83.

Tassinari CA, Cantalupo G, Rios-Pohl L, Della Giustina E, Rubboli G. Encephalopathy with status epilepticus during slow sleep: "the Penelope syndrome". *Epilepsia* 2009;50(7):4–8.

Tassinari CA, Cantalupo G, Rubboli G. Focal ESES as a selective focal brain dysfunction: a challenge for clinicians, an opportunity for cognitive neuroscientists. *Epileptic Disord* 2015;17(3):345–7.

Tassinari CA, Dravet C, Roger J. Encephalopathy related to electrical status epilepticus during slow sleep. *Electroenceph clin Neurophysiol* 1977;43:529–30.

Tassinari CA, Rubboli G, Volpi L, Billard C, Bureau M. Electrical status epilepticus during slow sleep (ESES or CSWS) including acquired epileptic aphasia (Landau-Kleffner syndrome). In: *epileptic syndromes in infancy, childhood and adolescence*. 4th Ed. Rodger J, Bureau M, Dravet C, Genton P, Tassinari CA, Wolf P. Montrouge: John Libbey Eurotext Ltd; 2005. p. 295–314.

Tassinari CA, Rubboli G, Volpi L, et al. Encephalopathy with electrical status epilepticus during slow sleep or ESES syndrome including the acquired aphasia. *Clin Neurophysiol* 2000;111(2):S94–102.

Tassinari CA, Rubboli G. Cognition and paroxysmal EEG activities: from a single spike to electrical status epilepticus during sleep. *Epilepsia* 2006;47(2):40–3.

Tassinari CA, Rubboli G. Encephalopathy related to Status Epilepticus during slow Sleep : current concepts and future directions. In: Encephalopathy related to Status Epilepticus during slow Sleep: linking epilepsy, sleep disruption and cognitive impairment. Rubboli G, Tassinari CA, editors. Montrouge: John Libbey Eurotext; 2020. p. 99–103.

Tassinari CA, Terrano G, Capocchi G, et al. Epileptic seizures during sleep in children. In: *Epilepsy, The 8th international symposium*. Penry JK. New York: Raven Press; 1977. p. 345–54.

Tassinari CA. The problems of continuous spikes and waves during slow sleep or electrical status epilepticus during slow sleep today. In: *Continuous spikes and waves during slow sleep*. Beaumanoir A, Bureau M, Deonna T, Mira L, Tassinari CA. London: John Libbey; 1995. p. 251–5.

Terzano MG, Parrino L, Spaggiari MC, Barusi R, Simeoni S. Discriminatory effect of cyclic alternating pattern in focal lesional and benign rolandic interictal spikes during sleep. *Epilepsia* 1991;32:616–28.

Tobler I. Phylogeny of sleep regulation. In: *Principles and practice of sleep medicine*. 3rd Ed. Kryger MH, Roth T, Dement WC. Philadelphia: Saunders; 2000. p. 72–81.

Tononi G, Cirelli C. Sleep and the price of plasticity: from synaptic and cellular homeostasis to memory consolidation and integration. *Neuron* 2014;81:12–34.

Tovia E, Goldberg-Stern H, Ben Zeev B, et al. The prevalence of atypical presentations and comorbidities of benign childhood epilepsy with centrotemporal spikes. *Epilepsia* 2011;52:1483–8.

Tsuru T, Mori M, Mizuguchi M, Momoi MY. Effects of high-dose intravenous corticosteroid therapy in Landau-Kleffner syndrome. *Pediatr Neurol* 2000;22:145–7.

Turner SJ, Morgan AT, Perez ER, Scheffer IE. New genes for focal epilepsies with speech and language disorders. *Curr Neurol Neurosci Rep* 2015;15:35.

Ujma PP, Simor P, Ferri R, et al. Increased interictal spike activity associated with transient slow-wave trains during non-rapid eye movement sleep: Increased IEDs in transient SW trains. *Sleep Biol Rhythms* 2015;13:155–62.

Urbain C, Di Vincenzo T, Peigneux P, Van Bogaert P. Is sleep-related consolidation impaired in focal idiopathic epilepsies of childhood? A pilot study. *Epilepsy Behav* 2011;22:380–4.

Urbain C, Galer S, Van Bogaert P, Peigneux P. Pathophysiology of sleep-dependent memory consolidation processes in children. *Int J Psychophysiol* 2013;89:273–83.

Vaags AK, Bowdin S, Smith ML, et al. Absent CNKSR2 causes seizures and intellectual., attention, and language deficits. *Ann Neurol* 2014;76(5):758–64.

Van Bogaert P, Urbain C, Galer S, et al. Impact of focal interictal epileptiform discharges on behaviour and cognition in children. *Neurophysiol Clin* 2012;42:53–8.

van Bogaert P. Epileptic encephalopathy with continuous spike-waves during slow-wave sleep including Landau-Kleffner syndrome: what determines outcome? In: *Outcome of childhood epilepsies*. Arts WF, Arzimanoglou A, Brouwer OF, Camfield C, Camfield P. Paris: John Libbey Eurotext; 2013. p. 141–8.

van den Munckhof B, Alderweireld C, Davelaar S, et al. Treatment of electrical status epilepticus in sleep: Clinical and EEG characteristics and response to 147 treatments in 47 patients. *Eur J Paediatr Neurol* 2018;22(1):64–71.

van den Munckhof B, de Vries EE, Braun KP, et al. Serum inflammatory mediators correlate with disease activity in electrical status epilepticus in sleep (ESES) syndrome. *Epilepsia* 2016;57(2):e45–50.

van den Munckhof B, van Dee V, Sagi L, et al. Treatment of electrical status epilepticus in sleep: a pooled analysis of 575 cases. *Epilepsia* 2015;56(11):1738–46.

Van Hirtum-Das M, Licht EA, Koh S, et al. Children with ESES: variability in the syndrome. *Epilepsy Res* 2006;70(S1):S248–58.

Van Hirtum-Das M, Licht EA, Koh S, Wu JY, Shields WD, Sankar R. Children with ESES: variability in the syndrome. *Epilepsy Res* 2006;70(1):248–58.

Vanhatalo S, Palva JM, Holmes MD, Miller JW, Voipio J, Kaila K. Infraslow oscillations modulate excitability and interictal epileptic activity in the human cortex during sleep. *PNAS* 2004;101:5053–7.

Vaudano AE, Laufs H, Kiebel SJ, et al. Causal hierarchy within thalamo-cortical network in spike and wave discharges. *PLoS One* 2009;4(8):e6475.

Vears DF, Tsai MH, Sadleir LG, et al. Clinical genetic studies in benign childhood epilepsy with centrotemporal spikes. *Epilepsia* 2012;53(2):319–24.

Vega C, Sánchez Fernández I, Peters J, et al. Response to clobazam in continuous spike-wave during sleep. *Dev Med Child Neurol* 2018;60(3):283–9.

Veggiotti P, Beccaria F, Papalia G, Termine C, Piazza F, Lanzi G. Continuous spikes and waves during sleep in children with shunted hydrocephalus. *Childs Nerv Syst* 1998;14:188–94.

Veggiotti P, Bova S, Granocchio E, et al. Acquired epileptic frontal syndrome as long-term outcome in two children with CSWS. *Neurophysiol Clin* 2001;31:387–97.

Veggiotti P, Pera MC, Teutonico F, Brazzo D, Balottin U, Tassinari CA. Therapy of encephalopathy with status epilepticus during sleep (ESES/CSWS syndrome): an update. *Epileptic Disord* 2012;14(1):1–11.

Vermeulen MCM, Vander Heijden KB, Swaab H, Van Someren EJW. Sleep spindle characteristics and sleep architecture are associated with learning of executive functions in school-age children. *J Sleep Res* 2018;e12779.

Ville D, Chiron C, Laschet J, Dulac O. The ketogenic diet can be used successfully in combination with corticosteroids for epileptic encephalopathies. *Epilepsy Behav* 2015;48:61–5.

von Stülpnagel C, Ensslen M, Møller RS, et al. Epilepsy in patients with GRIN2A alterations: Genetics, neurodevelopment, epileptic phenotype and response to anticonvulsive drugs. *Eur J Paediatr Neurol* 2017;21(3):530–41.

Vrielynck P, Marique P, Ghariani S, et al. Topiramate in childhood epileptic encephalopathy with continuous spike-waves during sleep: a retrospective study of 21 cases. *Eur J Paediatr Neurol* 2017;21(2):305–11.

Vyazovskiy VV, Cirelli C, Pfister-Genskow M, Faraguna U, Tononi G. Molecular and electrophysiological evidence for net synaptic potentiation in wake and depression in sleep. *Nat Neurosci* 2008;11:200–8.

Vyazovskiy VV, Olcese U, Lazimy YM, et al. Cortical firing and sleep homeostasis. *Neuron* 2009;63:865–78.

Vyazovskiy VV, Riedner BA, Cirelli C, Tononi G. Sleep homeostasis and cortical synchronization: II. A local field potential study of sleep slow waves in the rat. *Sleep* 2007;30:1631–42.

Walker L, Sills GJ. Inflammation and epilepsy: the foundations for a new therapeutic approach in epilepsy? *Epilepsy Curr* 2012;12:8–12.

Walker MP, Brakefield T, Morgan A, Hobson JA, Stickgold R. Practice with sleep makes perfect: sleep-dependent motor skill learning. *Neuron* 2002;35:205–11.

Wang S-B, Weng W-C, Fan P-C, Lee W-T. Levetiracetam in continuous spike waves during slow-wave sleep syndrome. *Pediatr Neurol* 2008;39:85–90.

Wasterlain CG, Fujikawa DG, Penix L, Sankar R. Pathophysiological mechanisms of brain damage from status epilepticus. *Epilepsia* 1993;34:S37–53.

Weber AB, Albert DV, Yin H, Held TP, Patel AD. Diagnosis of electrical status epilepticus during slow-wave sleep with 100 seconds of sleep. *J Clin Neurophysiol* 2017;34:65–8.

Wilhelm I, Kurth S, Ringli M, et al. Sleep slow-wave activity reveals developmental changes in experience-dependent plasticity. *J Neurosci* 2014;34:12568–75.

Wilson RB, Eliyan Y, Sankar R, Hussain SA. Amantadine: a new treatment for refractory electrical status epilepticus in sleep. *Epilepsy Behav* 2018;84:74–8.

Wirrell E, Ho AW-C, Hamiwka L. Sultiame therapy for continuous spike and wave in slow-wave sleep. *Pediatr Neurol* 2006;35:204–8.

Wolff M, Johannesen KM, Hedrich UBS, *et al*. Genetic and phenotypic heterogeneity suggest therapeutic implications in *SCN2A*-related disorders. *Brain* 2017;140:1316–36.

Wyllie E, Lachhwani DK, Gupta A, *et al*. Successful surgery for epilepsy due to early brain lesions despite generalized EEG findings. *Neurology* 2007;69:389–97.

Yuan H, Hansen KB, Zhang J, *et al*. Functional analysis of a de novo *GRIN2A* missense mutation associated with early-onset epileptic encephalopathy. *Nat Commun* 2014;5:3251.

Zanni G, Barresi S, Cohen R, *et al*. A novel mutation in the endosomal Na+/H+ exchanger NHE6 (SLC9A6) causes Christianson syndrome with electrical status epilepticus during slow-wave sleep (ESES). *Epilepsy Res* 2014;108(4):811–5.

Zubler F, Rubino A, Lo Russo G, Schindler K, Nobili L. Correlating interictal spikes with sigma and delta dynamics during non-rapid-eye-movement-sleep. *Front Neurol* 2017;8:288.

Achevé d'imprimer en novembre 2019 par Corlet Imprimeur — 14110 Condé-en-Normandie
Dépôt légal : novembre 2019 — N° d'imprimeur : 19110325 — *Imprimé en France*